The All-in-One Weight Loss Bible 2019

Transform Your Body with the Best
Intermittent Fasting, Ketogenic, Paleo, Vegan,
Keto Diet and Meal Plan Strategies of 2019
(Beginners Guide)

Written by Hannah Bedrosian

© Copyright 2019 Hannah Bedrosian - All rights reserved.

The content contained within this book may not be reproduced, duplicated or transmitted without direct written permission from the author or the publisher.

Under no circumstances will any blame or legal responsibility be held against the publisher, or author, for any damages, reparation, or monetary loss due to the information contained within this book. Either directly or indirectly.

<u>Legal Notice:</u>

This book is copyright protected. This book is only for personal use. You cannot amend, distribute, sell, use, quote or paraphrase any part, or the content within this book, without the consent of the author or publisher.

<u>Disclaimer Notice:</u>

Please note the information contained within this document is for educational and entertainment purposes only. All effort has been executed to present accurate, up to date, and reliable, complete information. No warranties of any kind are declared or implied. Readers acknowledge that the author is not engaging in the rendering of legal, financial, medical or professional advice. The content within this book has been derived from various sources. Please consult a licensed professional before attempting any techniques outlined in this book.

By reading this document, the reader agrees that under no circumstances is the author responsible for any losses, direct or indirect, which are incurred as a result of the use of information contained within this document, including, but not limited to, — errors, omissions, or inaccuracies.

Table Of Contents

Introduction 13

Chapter 1: Weight and your health 17

    Signs you need to start your weight loss and management journey 18

Chapter 2: Nutrition and weight loss management 24

    Understanding where you are 27

    Handling hunger 29

    Solving your diet puzzle 30

    A high fiber diet 31

    The fluids 32

    Some helpful tips 34

    Meal Plan 38

    Exercise Plan 39

    Self-care Plan 39

Chapter 3: The Keto Diet for weight loss 42

    Background 42

How ketogenic diet works 43

Types of ketogenic diet 43

    Fasting Ketosis 44

    Nutritional ketosis 45

Benefits of the keto diet 47

Getting Started with the keto diet plan 50

Sample Keto recipes: A look into a day on keto diet 52

    Breakfast 52

    Mid-morning snack 53

    Lunch 53

    Early evening snack 53

    Dinner 54

    Dessert 54

    Bottom line 54

Chapter 4: The Paleo Diet 56

Background of the Paleo diet 56

So what can I eat on the Paleo diet? 58

How to know what is paleo and what is not ... 61

Paleo diet and weight loss: How it works 62

Common Paleo Misconceptions 64

Benefits of Paleo diet 66
- Improve your metabolism 66
- Reduce inflammation 66
- Extend longevity 67
- Enhanced vitality 67
- Enhanced fitness 67
- Improved gut health 68

Being Human: Paleo is more than just a diet 68

Paleo diet in action: How to do it 69

Common mistakes made while on paleo diet 72
- Sustainability 72
- Failing to eat enough food 72
- Recreating junk food as paleo 73

Things to avoid when working on losing weight with paleo diet 73
- Zero carbohydrates 73
- Too many calories 74
- Excess proteins 74
- Just avoid fats 74
- Overlooking lost nutrients 75

A sample 5-day paleo diet menu 75
   Day 1 75
   Day 2 76
   Day 3 76
   Day 4 77
   Day 5 77

Chapter 5: The Vegan Diet 80

So what is a vegan diet? 80

Types of vegan diets 80

Vegan diet and weight loss 82

Vegan diet, blood sugar and Type II Diabetes 83

Vegan diet and cardiovascular health 84

Foods to avoid while on a vegan diet 85

Foods to eat while on a vegan diet 86

Risks and how to minimize them 89

A one-week vegan sample menu 92
   Monday 92
   Tuesday 93
   Wednesday 94
   Thursday 94

Friday 95

Saturday 95

Sunday 96

Eating out as a vegan 96

Some healthy vegan snacks 98

Chapter 6: Low Carbohydrate Diet 101

Purpose of low carb diet 101

Why you might take to a low carb diet 101

Low carbohydrate diet details 102

Typical foods in the low carb diet 105

Other health benefits of low carb diets 107

Low carb diet: what to drink 111

A simple one-week low carbohydrate menu . 113

Monday 113

Tuesday 114

Wednesday 114

Thursday 115

Friday 115

Saturday 116

Sunday 116

Healthy, low carbohydrate snacks 117

Eating at restaurants 118

A simple low carbohydrate shopping list 118

Chapter 7: Weight Loss and Fasting 122

So what is intermittent fasting? 122

So why fast? 124

Intermittent fasting as a powerful tool for your weight loss 126

Types of intermittent fasting 127

How to lose weight with intermittent fasting 128

Intermittent fasting and your hormones 128

Succeeding with intermittent fasting 131

Six popular ways to do intermittent fasting. 132

Chapter 8: Weight Loss and Exercise 138

Cardiovascular exercises and weight loss 142

Ten best cardio exercises for weight loss 143

How to sprint away from calories 152

Helpful tips for cardio exercises 153

How cardio can help you lose weight 154

The best cardio exercises 156

Weight lifting and weight loss 162

The best weight lifting exercises for weight loss 166

    Warming up 167

    Basic bodyweight workout 168

    Beast mode bodyweight exercises 169

    Classic gym circuit 170

    Tabata 171

    Battle ropes 174

    Killer kettlebells 174

    TRX training 176

    Metabolic strength 178

    Try-a-Tri 179

High Intensity Interval Training (HIIT) for Weight Loss 179

How to ensure that you are getting HIIT right 182

Getting started with HIIT 185

Benefits of HIIT 186

Top 10 HIIT workouts for weight loss 191

Chapter 9: Sports and Weight Loss 198

The 9 best sports that can accelerate your weight loss 198

    Individual sports 199

Team sports for weight loss 202

Chapter 10: Lifestyle adoption for weight loss, yoga, meditation, and Pilates. 205

    Yoga and weight loss 205

    Yoga and Mindfulness 205

    Yoga and better sleep 207

    Yoga and calorie burning 208

    Best yoga poses for weight loss 211

Meditation and weight loss 214

    What's the connection between meditation and weight loss? 215

    How can meditation help when diet and exercise don't seem to be working? 216

    How can you make sure meditation works for you? 218

What should you expect from doing guided meditation for weight loss? 220
Are there limitations to using meditation techniques for weight loss? 220
Meditation techniques for weight loss 221

Chapter 11: Pilates and weight loss 223
Tips for weight loss 235

Conclusion 237

Introduction

People opt for weight loss management for a number of reasons. Some people lose weight in preparation for the swimsuit season while others do so in preparation for a wedding. Yet, others lose weight to get in shape for a high school reunion. These are short-term motivations that rarely last after the intended event. There are also social reasons for losing weight, like shedding a few pounds because you want to look attractive to your partner. Whatever the motivation, anyone seeking long-term weight management must start by finding a reason that is important to them and not to other people.

To most people, improved health is one of the best motivations for lifestyle adjustment, and that is what this eBook will focus on: healthy, practical, and sustainable approaches to weight management.

Healthy weight management has nothing to with slim-down shakes or miracle pills. Rather, it takes work, time, and commitment. Clearly, the weight you are trying to lose did not show up overnight, and it is certainly going to take time to burn off. A healthy pace of weight loss is about 1-2 pounds per week. The rewards of a healthy lifestyle change can be phenomenal, with its effects on different aspects of your life. Making a conscious decision to embrace a healthy lifestyle will not just help you fit those skinny jeans, it will also let you set a great example for your kids that they can follow into adulthood. It will help you have a positive outlook as you go about your daily routines. It will equip you with the endurance you need to do the things you love for longer without running out of energy. It will boost your mood and self-esteem. And yes, it will save you money.

Weight management is never complicated. This eBook will show you that exercise and healthy eating are about finding the right balance – not consuming more calories than you can burn in a day at your present activity level. And you do not have to subscribe to a diet plan or buy premade foods. While some people reap great results from participating in support groups, nearly everyone is able to lose and sustain long-term weight loss without enrolling in any program.

Whether you enroll in a support group or not entirely depends on your needs and personality. However, if you feel this is something you cannot afford, or if you feel you will not have the time to attend meetings, or if social interactions are not quite your thing, then there is genuinely no reason to join one.

On the other hand, if you enjoy being around other people who share in the same experiences as you, or if you appreciate the idea of setting aside a day and time to join a group and weigh in for accountability purposes, or if you have the time and money, then you might find support groups tremendously helpful. However, there is a limit to how far support groups can go as far as your weight management is concerned. They will not make up your mind. They will not make you get out and exercise when you do not want to. They will not convince you to give up the mystery meat hot dog for the turkey sandwich. Bottomline: you will still have to have your own commitment and resolve every single day.

Long-term weight loss requires a complete lifestyle change. Of course, there will be moments of discomfort. There are days when you will want to give up. However, it is important to appreciate all the challenges on your weight loss path so you can handle them effectively. Remember, you will not make long-term changes unless you are willing to face and conquer the challenges on your path.

Chapter 1: Weight and your health

Excess weight is not just about your appearance. There is more to your weight than being unable to fit into your wedding dress, feel sexy in a swimsuit, or feel unattractive. Excess weight has serious health ramifications. Most folks appreciate that being overweight can put their health at risk. Unfortunately, sometimes it takes a rude awakening to make them understand just how dangerous being overweight can be. Not only will excess weight inhibit your mobility and the ability to do the things you enjoy, it also puts an undue burden on your organs. Here are some of the diseases associated with obesity or overweight: Type 2 diabetes, high cholesterol, coronary heart disease, stroke, gallbladder diseases, high blood pressure, osteoarthritis, some forms of cancer, sleep apnea and breathing difficulties, back and joint problems, pregnancy complications, and depression/ low self-esteem.

A recent Swedish study links obesity to Alzheimer's disease.

The weight loss and weight management journey: What you need to know before getting started.

If you want to shed weight and keep it at bay, and without interrupting your life, it is really prudent that you start with the key fundamentals of successful weight management. You do not have to make the journey harder than it needs to be by starting with a diet plan that requires you to eat like a caveman, or eliminate a set of foods that you enjoy.

Weight loss and management requires deliberate effort, but it should not feel like some form of punishment.

Signs you need to start your weight loss and management journey

Sometimes, weight gain can be so slow that you may not notice. Or, you just do not want to think about it presently. Maybe you have so much to do that you tell yourself you will eat healthy tomorrow or start working out in a few weeks' time. And then it happens, you wake up one morning and you cannot believe what you are seeing on the mirror. To get guesswork out of the way, here are a few signs and symptoms that it may be the right time to lose weight.

You can feel it!

You probably have a strong feeling when you need to shed some pounds. Let's face it – we often have the answers. All we need is the willingness to face the truth. Yes, admitting that you have gained weight can be tough; however, taking stock of where you are presently and deciding to begin your weight loss journey can get rid of a lot of stress and mental baggage you did not even know you were walking around with.

You find exercise a little bit challenging

If you do not wish to hit the gym because you are self-conscious about your extra-weight, or when you find exercising too strenuous because of your weight, these are telltale signs that it is about time you started shedding those extra pounds. If you are obese, workouts can sometimes seem an obstacle rather than a solution. Whatever challenges you are facing, sedentary lifestyle, obesity, muscle weakness, or lack of cardiovascular fitness, you can overcome them if you decide to. All you need to do is get started with something – chair exercises, walking, or swimming. Just start something.

Laboratory results indicate that you have hypertension and cholesterol and you are told you are almost diabetic

Excess fat, specifically belly fat, can increase your risk of developing type 2 diabetes and/or cardiovascular disease, and result in high cholesterol as well as hypertension. The good news is weight loss can bring down these numbers to healthy levels. The National Heart, Blood and Lung Institute report that inactive folks are two times more likely to develop cardiovascular complications than those who live an active lifestyle. When you lose weight, you can avoid a range of risks associated with these health complications. It may also help you avoid medications.

You snore

Excess weight can cause obstructive sleep apnea, a disorder characterized by non-rhythmic breathing during sleep. Loud gasping-like snoring is a symptom of sleep apnea. The disorder can result in decreased oxygen levels in the blood and can interfere with your sleep throughout the night. Excess weight and obesity is one of the most common causes of obstructive sleep apnea. If you feel tired most days and are told you snore loudly at night, chances are you have sleep apnea. Shed some pounds and you will not have to visit a sleep specialist.

You consistently gain several pounds every year

Do you consistently gain a few pounds each year? If your weight is steadily increasing, consider starting your weight loss journey.

You have painful joints

If your back, knees, and hips ache, it is probably due to the extra weight that you are carrying around. Excess weight exerts pressure on your joints and can wear down the tissue around these areas of the body, making your joints ache while moving.

You are full of excuses

Folks are quite great at denial and cooking excuses to avoid confronting the reality. If you spend a lot of time and energy explaining to yourself and friends why you are overweight, why you never exercise or how you detest healthy eating, all these excuses could be a sign that you need to make some changes.

You get winded scaling the stairs

If you get exhausted walking up the stairs or performing routine chores, it could be a sign that you are gaining weight. The National Institute of

Health report that your respiratory capacity decreases as you gain weight. Breathlessness is often linked to inactivity, a sign that your lungs and heart are not getting the exercise they need to optimally function.

Your clothes no longer fit

Oh, those skinny jeans you have had forever. If they are extremely tight, or no longer fit, it is time to lose weight.

Your numbers are off

If you have an elevated body mass index (BMI) and your waist is more than 35 inches, measured over your hip bones) consider shedding some pounds. BMI is the measure of your body fat based on weight and height and you can use it to gauge when you are sliding into obesity.

Chapter 2: Nutrition and weight loss management

Nutrition is, without doubt, the single most important factor in your weight loss management and healthy living journey. As such, it is important that you understand the importance of proper nutrition. Truth is, everyone loves to eat, and in our convenience-filled world, there is no such shortage of choices.

Sometimes, when thinking about healthy eating, you might want to think about the environment in which your body was original meant to live in: ideally, you are meant to exist on the verge of starvation, and you are perfectly equipped to make great use of berries, leaves, plants, nuts and an occasional diet of meat. And just in case your body is not able to exhaust the energy you consume each day in food, you have a wonderful energy storage mechanism called fat. Some body fat is essential for keeping you healthy, so you should not be striving for 0% body fat.

Most folks in developed nations no longer grapple with life-threatening hunger, but the daily array of choices combined with a first-world lifestyle is a recipe for other health complications. When you sit at your desk for eight or more hours a day, working at your computer with a slumped posture, spending several hours commuting to and from work, and winding off your day watching TV, your body will start to pay the price. Then you bring in additional scheduling challenges like taking kids to ballet lessons, football practice, and flute practice, and you are caught up in the modern lifestyle, a never-ending rat-race with very limited motion and lack of time for the essentials of life like workout habits and healthy eating.

When you start to notice the fruits of these lifestyle habits, either because your doctor has raised the red flag and warned you to shed a few pounds, or when your clothes no longer fit, you will be tempted to look for the easy way out. Those "miracle diet shakes" that miraculously rev up your metabolism, letting you burn more calories while making no changes to your lifestyle at all. Or, you have probably heard about the "body flush" diet – drinking lots of water while eating nothing to help "cleanse" your system.

There is no such thing as no-carb diet, high-carb diet, or even hot-dog diet. When you begin to focus on these "miracle" solutions, your head will most likely begin to swim. Nutrition is not as complicated as most marketers would want you to believe. Nutrition is easy, pure common sense that comprises of basic concepts that you probably already know – the kind of things your mom probably told you at the dining room table.

Here is the truth: there is no miracle weight loss shake. Any healthy weight loss program must come with a calorie deficit component, or burning more energy from the food you consume. To lose one pound, you need to burn 3500 calories. For most folks, taking in 250 calories per day and burning around 250 more creates a manageable deficit of 500 calories per day, and over the course of one week, you can lose one pound with this approach. One pound may seem insignificant, but you need to keep this number in perspective. How long did it take you to add the pounds you are trying to shed? If you gained five pounds in a week while on vacation, you are better off losing it in a month. If you gained 30 pounds while pregnant, keep in mind that it took you 9 months to gain weight, and it could take nearly the same amount of time to lose it. However, if you have lost focus on your weight and health for decades, and you realize you are 40 pounds or more above a healthy weight, then you need to be patient and understand that you will not lose all the weight overnight. Keep in mind that any kind of progress towards a healthy lifestyle is an important progress. In nutrition, just like with other aspects of life, baby steps are easier to adjust to than those enormous, large-scale life adjustments.

Understanding where you are

According to experts, one of the best ways to start

your weight loss journey is to get a clear idea of where you are currently. Pay attention to what you are eating and doing compared to some fundamental guidelines. Experts advise keeping a formal journal for a couple of days in which you note down everything you eat. You may take advantage of online nutritional labels and food calculators to get a precise idea of the calories in the food you take. The information for some of your favorite snacks may actually shock you.

Food journals are wonderful tools, but if you are willing to take advantage of them to make meaningful changes to your life. To achieve this, once you have kept track of all the foods you have eaten for a couple of days, take a serious study of your journal, as well as on the calorie and fat counts. With knowledge of the calorie cost of each food, it becomes easy to determine which one you can give up with ease without getting deprived. For most folks, there is really no reason to overhaul your diet from one day to the next. Start by looking out for the simple changes: keep in mind, if you consume 250 calories less and spend 250 calories more in the form of workouts, you could lose about one pound in a week. After a couple of weeks, you can identify another high-calorie favorite that you can drop for a healthier alternative.

Handling hunger

Most folks cringe at the word "diet" for fear of feeling grumpy and hungry all the time. However, experts say starving yourself is absolutely the wrong way around. In fact, experts recommend eating at least three meals per day, if not more. After all, it is a lot easier to resist a Quarter Pounder when you have already had a handful of fruits and nuts. Frequent small portions also give you a chance to ensure that you are getting a wide array of foods that include high-fiber foods. Just like your parents used to tell you: eat your vegetables, and yes, your breakfast is the most important meal of the day. If you are the type that often feels hungry on the days you skip breakfast, consider taking a protein and whole grain-rich breakfast. Simple carbohydrates like those present in sugary cereals or plain white bagels tend to burn off quite quickly. However, an egg-white omelet, or a bowl of oatmeal and fruits and a tablespoon of chopped almonds will certainly take your system longer to digest.

Solving your diet puzzle

Every week, it seems, comes with a new diet fad. Tabloids are filled with celebrities losing X pounds in three weeks with the pomegranate plan, and the next thing you notice, everyone you know is on the pomegranate plan, and asking you to join the bandwagon too.

Experts caution against jumping into these popular diets. Of course, you may realize some success with them, but this is usually short-lived. They often ignore important nutrients by asking you to completely give up certain foods. Additionally, certain plans can be dangerous if you have an underlying medical condition. For instance, some liquid or fasting diets can be dangerous for folks with sugar control issues or diabetes.

If you love the idea of a more formalized diet plan, then consider one from a reputable health-affiliated organization like the American Dietetic Association, the American Heart Association, or from a registered dietitian.

A high fiber diet

When talking about "high-fiber diet," the first thing that comes into most folks' minds is a bowl of bark-like bran cereal, or a fiber beverage mix that you stir into a glass of water, that tastes more like sand! While these items have their place in the world, for most folks, increasing fiber in the diet is just a matter of eating fresh fruits and a few more vegetables.

According to experts, a high fiber diet will not only help your gut function properly, which is key to preventing diverticulitis (a painful intestinal disorder) but also helps prevent some forms of colon cancers and cardiovascular conditions because some fibers help scrub the walls of the intestines while others play a role in lowering the body's cholesterol levels. Fibers also let you feel full and satisfied after your meal, plus they take much longer to digest. This leaves you feeling full long after your meals.

Your body cannot break down and utilize the fiber itself, so this is a smart way of adding to your food volume without increasing your calorie intake. Some of the best sources of fiber include greens, fruits, and vegetables. Not only is it easy for the body to handle these, you will also get the nutrients you need.

The fluids

Besides what you eat in a day, nutrition also has a lot to do with what you drink. Water is the best fluid for your body. It is calorie-free and essential for your body's physiological functions. Other beneficial fluids include juices, but these can be calorie-rich. A modest amount of tea and coffee is also good.

Failing to drink enough fluids will, of course, cause dehydration, which will increase your vulnerability to a myriad of health complications like constipation and heat stroke. Sometimes, your body will tell your brain that "I'm hungry" when in the real sense it is just thirsty. Staying well hydrated can prevent such a situation.

The more you work out the more you will need to be hydrated. Professional athletes pay a lot of attention to their fluid levels, but for the average folk, it is enough to be aware that it is imperative to understand that you need to be adequately hydrated at all times, especially before and after your exercises.

Some fluids can work against your weight loss campaign, like full-sugar sodas, that bring no nutritional benefits but just pile up your calorie levels. Diet sodas with artificial sweeteners do not come with extra calories, but most are caffeinated, which actually drain water from your body.

Sports drinks can be helpful, especially if you are exercising intensely for over an hour at a time. Even then, low calorie sports drinks are excellent. If you are working in the low to moderate range for less than an hour at a time, plain tap water is a wonderful calorie-free way to remain hydrated during your workout.

Some helpful tips

While starting a diet to lose weight and improve your health is a worthy goal, the truth is it can be a bit overwhelming. Challenges are bound to happen when you start a new initiative, especially when it involves something you get to do multiple times each day – like eating and drinking.

Still, as long as you do not make radical changes all at once, you can realize your weight loss goals. Here are helpful tips to get started in your weight loss journey as a newbie and stay on course for the long haul.

- Get the right mindset

When it comes to weight loss, most folks automatically assume that diet and exercise are the key drivers for success. While these factors play a crucial role in your weight loss campaign, there is another ingredient that is equally, if not more, important: your state of mind. Studies show that self-efficacy plays a vital role in your ability to successfully manage weight. In other words, the more you have confidence in yourself and your ability to follow through with your weight loss plan, the more pounds you are likely to shed. Here are a couple of ways you can build self-efficacy when it comes to weight loss.

- Determine your "why"

If you acquire the right mindset and have faith in your weight loss campaign, you are going to have to go further than the generic "I should lose weight" resolution. Of course, wanting to lose weight is great. However, finding a deeper meaning to your weight loss effort will help put your mind on the right track. Here are examples of meaningful reasons why you might want to lose weight:

- So you can gain more energy and mental clarity

- To boost your self confidence

- To manage or reverse diabetes and obesity

- To set a good example for your kids

- Be prepared to make mistakes

One of the greatest setbacks for beginners on their weight loss journey is getting in with an "all-or-nothing" mindset. Acquiring self-efficacy has nothing to do with believing that you will be perfect. No, not at all! Rather, self-efficacy has to do with believing you will achieve your goals regardless of inevitable setbacks.

You are setting yourself up for failure when you do not make room for mistakes. A time will come when you will find yourself eating something you should not, skip your exercise, or even fall off track for a couple of days. Preparing yourself for this beforehand and believing in your ability to bounce back is key to setting up yourself for long-term weight loss success.

- Be clear about what motivates you

Let's be honest, weight loss is not an easy journey. There will be times, probably many, when you will not feel like preparing your healthy food or exercising. You have to figure out what helps you push through those challenging times. Part of your motivation may include remembering your weight loss "whys."

- Come up with a plan

Alan Lakein was right when he said failing to plan is planning to fail.

It is pretty easy to come up with excuses as to why you "just cannot" today. You neither have healthy food at home nor time to cook, or you are just too busy to create time for exercise. Of course, there will be times when life will get in the way, and that is perfectly fine. But most often, excuses will abound when you do not have a plan in place in the first place.

Meal Plan

Nutrition plays a crucial role in your weight loss effort. You need to nourish your body with proper nutrients to burn the fats, build muscles, and maintain your energy levels. But without a plan in place, you are likely to fall off track with your eating habits. Here are a few tips for a simple, yet effective, meal planning:

- For easy access to your recipes, find a space to store them like binders, apps, or Pinterest board

- Save on time and money by cooking weekly meals that have the same ingredients

- Prepare large dishes to make for leftovers

- Create a list of the meals you would love to

make a week ahead

- Keep your kitchen well stocked with healthy options

Exercise Plan

As you already know, exercise is another crucial part of your weight loss campaign. Physical activity helps burn fat, maintain a healthy muscle mass, keep your heart active, and boost your body's calorie-burning ability. However, without a workout plan, it is easy to leave exercise out of your routine. Your workouts should be treated like an appointment. Consider scheduling them into your daily routine so you can set aside the time for exercises.

Self-care Plan

Yes, you read that right! Self-care is just as critical, perhaps even more so than your exercise and diet plans. Schedule some time just for you. This will help you avoid burnouts. You could spend this time reading your favorite book, relaxing with a cup of tea, enjoying a hot bath, whatever gets you relaxed, set some time to take the edge off at least once every week.

- Write down your starting points

Tracking your weight loss progress is going to be your greatest source of motivation. When you begin to notice changes, you will want to keep going. However, to track this progress, you will need to know where you are starting at. Note down your starting measurements, that way you will be able to monitor how much you are changing.

Here are important things to note down:

- your weight

- your measurements (waist, chest, and hips)

- a list of how you are feeling (cravings and mood, energy levels, hunger)

- before and after pictures

- Make it enjoyable

The number one advice for everyone seeking to lose weight is to make the journey enjoyable. Never stress over a single calorie. Never beat up yourself if you fall for a bar of chocolate or if you skip your exercise. Being too rigid is a perfect way to burn out and lose interest. In fact, studies indicate that most people who lose weight gain most of it back due to extreme dieting or exercising. So take things easy and enjoy your weight loss journey. Accept and take lessons from your mistakes. Be kind to yourself when things do not go as planned. Reward yourself when you accomplish even the smallest goals. This is how you make your weight loss journey a lifestyle that you love.

Chapter 3: The Keto Diet for weight loss

Background

The ketogenic, commonly known as the keto diet, is a low carbohydrate, fat-rich eating plan that has been around for centuries to manage specific medical conditions. The keto diet was used in the 19th century to manage diabetes. In the 1920s, it was used to treat epileptic children in situations where conventional medication was ineffective. This diet has also been tested and used to monitor settings for polycystic ovary syndrome, diabetes, Alzheimer's diseases, and certain forms of cancer.

However, in recent times, the ketogenic diet has gained considerable attention as an effective weight loss diet plan thanks to the low-carb diet craze, which began in the 1970s with the Atkins diet. The keto diet stands out for its exceptional high-fat content, usually 70% to 80%, with a moderate protein intake.

How ketogenic diet works

The logic of the ketogenic diet for weight loss and management is that you starve your body of glucose – the cells' main source of energy, which you obtain by eating carbohydrate foods, an alternative fuel known as ketones is generated from stored fat. The brain requires a lot of glucose, about 120 grams per day because it is not able to store glucose. When fasting, or when on a low carbohydrate diet, the body starts by pulling stored glucose from the liver and temporarily breaks down muscles to release glucose. Upon depleting glucose in the muscles, blood levels of a hormone called insulin decrease and the body begins to utilize fat as the primary source of fuel. The liver then produces ketone bodies from fat which is used in the absence of glucose.

Types of ketogenic diet

As already indicated, the ketogenic diet is designed to bring about ketosis, the breaking down of fat into ketones to allow the body to run on ketones in place of glucose. Ketosis can be brought about in a number of ways and thus the different variants of ketogenic diet.

Since the end goal of keto diets is the same, the different variants of the ketogenic diet do share a number of similarities, notably in being low in carbohydrate and high in dietary fat.

Fasting Ketosis

The idea of fasting has been around for centuries, and played a crucial role in the origins of the ketogenic diet. In fact, fasting has been praised by great philosophers like Socrates, Hippocrates, and Aristotle.

While fasting, depletion of glycogen (stored glucose) in the liver triggers chemical signals within the body to start burning more fat, resulting in the production of more ketones. As you continue with the fast, blood glucose continues to plummet, and the extent of ketogenesis increases as a result of the depletion of the TCA cycle intermediate oxaloacetate.

Fasting ketosis can have a range of health benefits and has been used to manage obesity as well as to induce ketosis before chemotherapy.

Nutritional ketosis

This variant of ketosis is induced by dietary modification. Nutritional ketosis can be subdivided into three subcategories:

- Carbohydrate restricted ketosis
- Supplemental ketosis
- Alcoholic ketosis

Carbohydrate ketosis

Carbohydrate-restricted ketosis has been around for decades. It is commonly used to achieve a state of ketosis, and typically results in an increase in ketones compared to an overnight fast. A high-fat, low-carbohydrate (usually 30 grams), and moderate intake of proteins is generally accepted as the best method of realizing carbohydrate-restricted ketosis. Carbohydrate ketosis is a long-term, sustainable weight loss approach that can provide a range of health benefits such as blood sugar, improved cognition, weight loss, and management of various health conditions.

Supplemental ketosis

Ketosis can also provide powerful therapeutic effects. However, the level of supplemental ketosis must be greater than that of fasting and carbohydrate-restricted ketosis. Supplemental ketosis can be used in combination with carbohydrate-restricted ketosis and has been applied over the years to manage or aid in treatment of metabolic disorders, neurological disorders like Alzheimer's disease, some forms of cancer, as well as diabetes. And since ketones are an alternative energy source, supplemental ketones are ideal for providing performance benefits to athletes.

Alcoholic ketosis

Alcohol ketoacidosis, commonly known as alcoholic ketosis or AKA, is technically classified as nutritional ketosis since it occurs as a result of dietary intervention. As the name suggests, this form of ketosis results from alcohol consumption and triggers an acidic internal environment caused by a sudden increase in ketone bodies. It is common in those who drink while under malnutrition. It is characterized by nausea, fatigue, vomiting, irregular breathing, and abdominal pain.

Benefits of the keto diet

Most diets come with only one benefit and that is weight loss. The problem with this being the sole benefit is that is becomes quite easy to fall through the cracks. Keto diet comes with multiple benefits due to how it changes the body's chemistry. Your body becomes much more efficient when it is powered by ketones as the primary source of fuel.

Here are some of the benefits of the keto diet

Weight loss

This, of course, remains the number one reason why most people opt for the keto diet. Since fat becomes a source of energy, your body embarks on actively burning fats for energy rather looking for glucose.

Appetite control

Something interesting happens when your diet is devoid of carbs. You notice that you are not as hungry as often, and you do not end up with persistent cravings that lure you into eating unintended foods. Most folks who opt for keto can combine it with intermittent fasting which gets them to eat only during certain periods of the day. This becomes possible because your stomach does not rumble about compelling you to reach for a donut.

Better mental focus

The problem with relying on carbs as your primary energy source is that they cause a rise and fall in your blood's sugar levels. And since the energy source is not consistent, it becomes hard for your brain to remain focused for an extended period of time. When you are on keto diet, your brain draws its energy from the ketones, which is a consistent source and this means that you can remain focused for long.

More energy

There is a limit to the amount of glycogen your body can store, and due to this, it is important that you consistently refuel if you want to keep your energy levels high. However, you already have plenty of fat to work with and you can store more fat, meaning that ketosis is an energy source that you will never deplete. This means that your energy levels will be high throughout the day.

Helps fight Type II Diabetes

Patients with Type II Diabetes usually suffer from high insulin production. Since ketogenic diet eliminates sugars from the diet, it tends to lower the HbA1c, and thus can effectively counter Type II Diabetes.

Lower blood pressure

Hypertension is a sign of future cardiovascular problems. Ketogenic diet does an excellent job of lowering blood pressure.

Getting Started with the keto diet plan

It is important that you have a keto food list:

Ready to step out and start stocking groceries? Hold on one minute. Go through your fridge, pantry, freezer, and those secret stashes under your bed and get rid of everything high in carbs. Of course, in the few days, you will crave for them – and badly so. That done, here are the staples that you should build your keto diet around.

- Fat-rich nuts and seeds like macadamia nuts, cashew nuts, pumpkin seeds
- Whole eggs
- Avocado
- Full-fat cheese
- Chicken thighs and legs
- Beef
- Vegetables like spinach, cabbage, asparagus, broccoli, bell pepper, and mushrooms
- Olive oil
- Pork rinds
- Heavy cream
- Salted butter
- Source cream
- Fatty fish like mackerel, salmon, anchovies, and salmon

- Bacon

Snack ideas include

- Cubed cheese
- Pork rinds
- Jerky
- Nuts and seeds
- Sugar free Jello
- Veggies and dip

Sample Keto recipes: A look into a day on keto diet

As an example of what a ketogenic diet may look like, here is a simple meal plan that you may try out:

Breakfast

- 1 cup of coffee blended with a tablespoon of butter and a dash of cinnamon
- 2 eggs cooked in a tablespoon of ghee or

butter

- ½ cup of cooked spinach in a tablespoon of coconut oil

Mid-morning snack

- 6 raspberries
- 6 macadamia nuts

Lunch

- Tuna salad made from 4-5 ounces of canned light tuna mixed with ¼ cup chopped celery, 2 tablespoons of mayonnaise, ¼ cup of chopped green apple, and black pepper or salt to taste – served over a cup of Romaine lettuce
- ½ cup of steamed green beans and 8-10 olives, topped with a mixture of ½ lemon and 1 tablespoon olive oil.

Early evening snack

½ avocado sprinkled with 1 tablespoon of

nutritional yeast or hemp seeds

Dinner

- 1 cup cauliflower roasted in 1 tablespoon hazelnut oil

- 8-12 ounces of cooked steak in 1 tablespoon of butter

Dessert

- 1 tablespoon crunchy salted almond butter sprinkled with a dash of cinnamon

- 1 ounce 90% dark chocolate

Bottom line

A ketogenic diet is an ideal option for folks who have had challenges losing weight with other methods. The exact combination of carbohydrate, fat, and protein needed to achieve the desired health benefits vary from individual to individual due to varying genetic makeups as well as body composition. Therefore, it is recommended that you consult with your physician or dietician before getting started with ketogenic diet so that you can be closely monitored for any biochemical changes after starting the diet plan, and create a plan that fits your current health conditions as well as prevent nutritional deficiencies or other health complications that may arise. Your dietician may also recommend guidelines on how to reintroduce carbohydrates into your diet once you have attained the desired weight loss.

Chapter 4: The Paleo Diet

Paleo diet is based on a very simple premise – if the caveman did not touch it, neither should you. So long to dairy products, refined sugars, grains and legumes (this is the era of pre-agricultural revolution), and hello to fish, meat, veggies, and fruits. The argument is that by avoiding modern-day foods like dairy and highly processed carbohydrates, you can push back or avoid "diseases of civilization" like cardiovascular conditions, Type II Diabetes, and shed some pounds too in the process. The foods you take, and quantity, depends on your goals as well as the specific Paleo program you are on.

Background of the Paleo diet

The Paleo diet, it is believed, began centuries ago in a cave. Probably in Africa.

The human body has evolved over millions of years, and man has only been eating grains and other foods since the agricultural revolution, which dates back to 10,000 years ago. While this might sound like a long time, it is really a tiny amount of time compared to how long man has been around this blue marble planet.

As it turns out, the human body is best suited for eating foods different from what we are accustomed to eating these days. The large amounts of sugars in processed foods that permeate modern diets just were never around when your great-great-great forefathers were roaming around throwing arrows and spears at saber tooth tigers.

And, since man has been feasting on processed grains since the arrival of the agricultural revolution, our bodies never quite gave up their caveman roots. And besides that, grains do not like to be eaten. There are tons of dangers associated with eating grains. Studies have shown that grains can hurt the immune system, damage the lining of your gut, and cause several other health complications. Simply put, things get messy when you eat grains.

The Paleo diet advocates eating like the ancient man, mostly feeding on fresh fruits, meat, eggs, vegetables, and nuts.

So what can I eat on the Paleo diet?

Great question! Here is a quick rundown of the foods that make up the Paleo diet. They are the foods your ancestors had access to on a regular basis.

- Lean meats – veal, beef, chicken, lamb, bison (try as much as you can to eat the grass-fed versions of these)

- Fish tilapia, bass, salmon

- Eggs

- Seafood

- Vegetables

- Fruits – especially berries and the less sugary ones

- Nuts – in moderation

- Natural oils

The point is, if a hunter-gatherer could not eat it 10,000 years ago, simply avoid it. And that means no to Oreos, Twinkies, or that breakfast cereal, sorry. There are tons of paleo foods out there for you, and they are pretty tasty. Oh, and if it contains chemicals that you just cannot pronounce, it is clearly not paleo... again, sorry!

Are grains on the list of paleo foods?

This is an easy one. NO.

What about dairy?

The quick answer is NO. The more complex answer is, "well, that depends."

Remember, there is no rule set for the paleo diet. Rather, paleo is more of a framework than a diet plan. Some liberal paleo dieters include fermented dairy products in their plans while more strict paleo dieters exclude milk completely, arguing that the caveman had no cows grazing around his cave. Whatever side of the spectrum you are on, the more processed a food is, the less paleo it is. That makes whole milk far better than 2% milk which, in turn, is better than skim milk.

How about yogurt, cheese, butter, and ice cream?

Another great question. With widespread cases of lactose intolerance, it is surprising that man continues to consume such high quantities of dairy. But as with carbs, dairy comes on a sliding scale. Here is a closer look.

Most folks widely consider grass-fed butter. It is a great source of fat and has some omega-3 to omega-6 fatty acid ratio, so having this in your diet occasionally is acceptable.

Yogurt falls in the grey area. The probiotics in yogurt help improve digestion and it is a traditional way of extending dairy's shelf life. The only drawback is the high sugar levels in most yogurts. Again, the rule is that the more processed a food is, the less paleo it is.

Cheese is another relatively safe form of dairy.

The fermentation process gets rid of most of the lactose that may be a problem to those with lactose intolerance.

Ice cream, however, is a no-go. You may treat yourself to it once in a while. But keep in mind that it has too much sugar to be a regular staple in your paleo diet.

Are legumes paleo?

A legume, for starters, is a pod fruit. Some of the common legumes you are probably familiar with include peas, beans, peanuts, lentils, clover, alfalfa, soy, carob, and lupins. It is important to understand that legumes are NOT paleo.

How to know what is paleo and what is not

Ideally, it is clear whether or not a food is paleo. Beef exists naturally in the form of cattle, so it is paleo. Ice cream, on the other hand, does not exist naturally in the world and it is processed by man, so it is clearly not paleo.

But sometimes, there is a fine line between paleo and non-paleo foods. For instance, it is easy to think peanuts are paleo because nuts are paleo. Unfortunately, peanuts are actually a legume, which make it non-paleo. You can also take advantage of free applications to know what is paleo and what is not.

Paleo diet and weight loss: How it works

The main reason most folks find paleo diet to be a very effective method for losing weight is that it turns your body from a carbohydrate-burning machine to a fat-burning machine.

Here is how paleo works (burning carbohydrates vs. burning fat)

Fats are your body's preferred source of energy. Fat is a slow burning fuel, and it is more efficient for powering your body. However, due to the amount of carbohydrates people consume, especially in the developed world, the body burns carbohydrates rather than fats. Thus, when you take in more carbohydrates than surpasses the energy you need, your body converts and stores surplus as fats "for later use."

Fortunately (or unfortunately, depending on how you see it), most folks will never be in danger of "starving." Most often, we never have to turn to our fat reservoirs of energy, so instead of burning the fat you are storing in your body, you simply add to it, over and over again. This explains why obesity is a rampant problem in the Western world.

The paleo diet confronts this through one simple approach: eliminating a lot of simple carbohydrates from your diet. When this happens, your body will no longer turn to cheap carbohydrates for energy supply, so it has to burn the stored fat. And that is great!

With the constant supply of cheap carbohydrates that your body would otherwise burn for energy, your blood sugar will drop and your insulin levels begin to regulate. Regulated insulin levels enable a process known as lipolysis. This is the process where your body releases triglycerides (fat stores) to be converted to energy. That sounds like a bunch of big words. Basically, this is what we are talking about: by cutting off cheap carbohydrates from your diet, the paleo diet allows your body to embark on a fat-burning mission. And this is how paleo diet helps you lose weight.

Common Paleo Misconceptions

Good carbohydrates vs. bad carbohydrates

So, are all carbohydrates no-go? No, not all carbs are bad. Some are clearly worse than others and there is certainly a sliding scale of carb badness.

It is easy to jump from "take fewer carbs" to "all carbs are a no-go." Again, there is a sliding scale. You have probably heard about simple carbohydrates and complex carbohydrates, and while these can be a little difficult to differentiate, basically, when it comes to carbs, the question you should be asking is how fast your body will burn the carbs you are eating into sugar.

Carbohydrates that are burnt fast are referred to as "simple carbs" (and you should avoid these), while carbohydrates that take longer to digest are referred to as "complex carbs" (and you can take these in moderation).

Simple carbohydrates break down faster than complex carbs, and this triggers bigger insulin response. Elevated insulin levels prevent your body from burning fat. This is the main reason you should avoid simple carbohydrates like pasta and white bread. Eating them is no different from munching straight sugar!

Isn't fat bad for you?

No, it is not. Well, not the way you have been made to believe. Most people think that fat should be shunned because the body gets it directly from the food and deposits it right onto the belly area, right? Well, that is not really how it happens.

As you probably already know, your body's preferred source of energy is actually fat. Yes, fat is a slow burning, longer lasting fuel than carbs. Because of this, when you stop taking in simple carbs and sugar day after day, your body will turn to body fat for energy – energy that was, otherwise, stored in your body in the form of fat. Remember, this energy remains unused as long as you are taking in more energy than you need in the form of sugar from simple carbohydrates.

Benefits of Paleo diet

Here are some of the amazing benefits of paleo diet.

Improve your metabolism

A recent study showed that a Paleolithic diet reduces the markers of metabolism syndrome as observed in diabetes, fasting blood glucose, waist circumference, as well as blood pressure and cholesterol.

Reduce inflammation

Findings from 11 different studies show that

paleo diet significantly reduces inflammation, especially in heart disease and Type II Diabetes patients.

Extend longevity

Paleolithic diet has been show to enhance longevity. According to the Journal of Nutrition, those who follow Paleo or Mediterranean diet plan tend to live longer.

Enhanced vitality

Paleo diet enhances an individual's blood sugar regulation, improves mineral and vitamin status, reduces weight and inflammation, and lowers the blood pressure.

Enhanced fitness

Beyond food, studies show that the paleo diet can reward you with a more active lifestyle. Those who are on a paleo diet plan, like the hunter-gatherer, are much more active than the average westerner with his sedentary lifestyle.

Improved gut health

A recent review of the effect of paleo on the human gut concluded that a Paleolithic diet can enhance healthier and more diverse gut bacteria.

Being Human: Paleo is more than just a diet

A paleo diet not only includes real food (veggies fruits, proteins, and healthy fats), it also encourages:

- Eating high-quality, seasonal, sustainable, nutrient-rich (such as organic and pastured meats, raw soaked seeds and nuts, non-GMO seasonal produce, and non-rancid fat and oils)

- Remaining hydrated with clean, spring or reverse osmosis water

- Integrating activity, play and primal, and functional movement like squats, pulls, pushes, lunging, walking, into your daily lifestyle.

- Restoring your energy through rest, leisure, and quality sleep

- Maintaining alertness

- Connecting

- Financial health and stability

- Mindful use of technology

Paleo diet in action: How to do it

Step 1: Eat real food

Simplified, put more emphasis on whole and minimally processed foods while avoiding heavily processed foods. Can you fish, hunt, or trap it? Can you pluck it from a tree or pull it from the ground? If your answer is yes then you are clearly on the right track.

Eat these:

- Veggies (for fiber and micronutrients)

- Fish, meat, fowl, and eggs

- Healthy fats
- Herbs and spices
- Roots and tubers
- Fruits in moderation
- Bone broths and fermented foods

So how long does it take to lose weight on the paleo diet?

Losing weight is not a walk in the park. And with grocery shelves full of processed junks with lots of unhealthy fats and refined sugars, weight loss becomes even more challenging. The right, and the best, way of losing weight is through healthy eating and regular exercise, including a complete lifestyle change.

Paleo diet helps you eat right by avoiding everything that was not around during the primal era. This avoidance is based on the premise that the early man never suffered from degenerative medical conditions that are rampant today such as obesity, diabetes, cardiovascular diseases, and certain forms of cancer.

As already mentioned, paleo diet involves eating fruits, meat, seafood, veggies, fish, eggs, and nuts. The meat cuts should only be derived from pasture-fed animals. Paleo diet eliminates grains, sugar, processed foods, potatoes, refined vegetable oils, and legumes from your diet.

Expected weight loss

It is important to note that paleo diet weight loss is not for everyone. That said, people on this diet experience significant weight loss in the first week. This is due to a loss in water weight as a result of reduction of carbs in the diet.

Depending on your starting weight, you can expect to lose anything from 5-11 pounds with paleo diet. However, after the first week, due to reduced water weight, weight loss slows down significantly. You may drop around two pounds per week until you reach a plateau or your desired weight.

Common mistakes made while on paleo diet

Sustainability

One of the most common mistakes dieters make when it comes to the paleo diet is sustainability. Most people focus on weight loss after which they do away with the diet and resume their usual unhealthy eating habit. On the contrary, this diet is designed to be a lifestyle change to avoid and keep common health concerns at bay. All adjustments you make to your diet should be sustainable in the long run.

Failing to eat enough food

Most paleo beginners make this mistake. When you are on paleo diet, you need to eat enough food to ensure that you are getting adequate carbohydrates and healthy fats. This is key if you want to maintain optimum performance throughout your day. Never starve yourself. Also, be certain that you eat whenever you are hungry without worrying about the time.

Recreating junk food as paleo

Some foods find their way into the paleo diet when they are not quite paleo. In fact, they will never aid your weight loss journey in any way. Foods like paleo cookies, paleo pancakes, paleo ice cream, paleo pizza, paleo candy, and similar foods are made using "paleo ingredients". However, they are not paleo and, therefore, do not belong anywhere near your paleo plate.

Things to avoid when working on losing weight with paleo diet

If you are on paleo diet to lose weight, then here are some of the things you need to keep off your menu:

Zero carbohydrates

By now, you already know there are healthy carbs and unhealthy ones. It is important to take small portions of healthy carbohydrates, just enough to nourish you with the energy you need for the day. It is important to understand that the paleo diet is not a zero carb diet. Be sure to make healthy portions of complex carbs like sweet potatoes and potatoes part of your diet.

Too many calories

Weight loss is all about cutting down your calorie intake. Therefore, if your calorie intake, whether from healthy foods or not, is more than your daily requirement, there will be storage of excess carbohydrates in the form of fats. Thus, ensure that you keep your calorie-consumption in check.

Excess proteins

You cannot have too many proteins in your paleo diet. The recommended protein levels should not be more than one-third of your plate.

Just avoid fats

Mono-saturated fats like the ones in healthy nuts are allowed in paleo diet. Also, ensure that your meat is only from pasture-fed animals. You can obtain fats from olive oil, avocado, seeds, nuts, and coconut oil: avoid such foods.

Overlooking lost nutrients

Foods most folks ignore but are part of the paleo diet include dairy, grains and legumes are nutritious, adding to your source of nutrients. If it important to check with your nutritionist if you are missing some nutrients so you can find a way of replacing them.

A sample 5-day paleo diet menu

Day 1

Breakfast

Prepare your favorite egg with sausage and a side of berries

Lunch

A bowl of garlic Cajun shrimp with spiralized zucchini

Dinner

Slow-cooker sweet potato chili with green chilies and ground beef or bison

Day 2

Breakfast

A bowl of gluten-free paleo porridge with pumpkin seeds, coconut, and chia seeds

Lunch

Cauliflower, broccoli, an orange salad with added shrimp or grilled chicken

Dinner

Thai wraps with ground chicken and Bibb lettuce

Day 3

Breakfast

Paleo pancakes prepared with coconut flour and added berries

Lunch

Roasted sweet potato vegetable salad with added chicken and crumbled bacon

Dinner

Ginger, beef, and broccoli stir-fry cooked in ghee

Day 4

Breakfast

Chorizo breakfast scrambled with eggs, veggies, gluten-free chorizo sausage, and herbs

Lunch

A paleo-friendly vegetable soup

Dinner

One-pan lemon chicken with garlic, asparagus, and herbs

Day 5

Breakfast

Italian spaghetti squash breakfast casserole with

salami, eggs, olives, and tomatoes.

Lunch

Paleo pinwheels with cashew cream cheese

Dinner

Slow-cooker Hawaiian shredded chicken with citrus and avocado served with lettuce wraps.

Bottom line

A paleo diet, also known as caveman diet, Stone Age diet, or the hunter-gatherer diet, is basically a dietary plan based on foods similar to what the cavemen ate in the Paleolithic era, prior to the agricultural revolution. The diet includes fruits, lean meats, vegetables, fish, seeds and nuts – foods that the caveman obtained by hunting and gathering. Dairy products, grains, and legumes are not part of this diet. Paleo diet is great for folks who want to shed extra pounds and maintain a healthy weight or are keen to plan their meals.

Hannah Bedrosian

Chapter 5: The Vegan Diet

Vegan diet has gained popularity in recent years for health, environmental, and ethical reasons. When done right, the vegan diet may yield multiple health benefits, including an improved blood sugar control, as well as a trimmer waistline. However, it is important to note that a diet that is exclusively based on plant foods may, in some cases, increase the risk of nutrient deficiency.

So what is a vegan diet?

A vegan lifestyle attempts to eliminate all forms of animal exploitation and cruelty, whether for clothing, food, or any other purpose. For this reason, the vegan diet is free of any form of animal products, including dairy, eggs, and meat. People opt for vegan diet for a myriad of reasons, from environmental and ethical concerns as well as from the desire to improve health.

Types of vegan diets

Vegan diet comes in a range of variations. Here are the most common ones:

- Whole food vegan diet

This vegan diet plan is based on a wide variety of whole plant foods like vegetables, fruits, legumes, whole grains, seeds, and nuts.

- Raw food vegan diet

This vegan diet is based on raw fruits, nuts, vegetables, seeds, and plant foods that are cooked at temperatures below 118 degrees F.

- 80/10/10

This raw-food vegan diet avoids fat-rich plants like avocado and nuts and roots for soft greens and raw fruits instead. It is also referred to as raw-food, law-fat vegan diet, or fruitarian diet.

- The starch solution

This low-fat, high-carbohydrate vegan diet shares similarities with the 80/10/10. However, it focuses on cooked starches like rice, potatoes, and corn in place of fruits.

- Raw till 4

This low-fat vegan diet also draws its inspiration from the 80/10/10 and starch solution. You can take raw foods until 4pm before opting for a cooked plant-based meal for dinner.

- The thrive diet

This is another raw-food vegan diet. Dieters consume plant-based foods whole that are either raw or minimally cooked at low temperatures.

- Junk-food vegan diet

This vegan diet lacks in whole plant food and instead relies heavily on the mock meats, fries, cheese, vegan desserts, and other heavily processed vegan foods.

Vegan diet and weight loss

Statistically, vegans tend to be thinner, usually

with a lower body mass index (BMI) than non-vegans. This could explain why folks are turning to vegan diets as a way of losing weight.

Part of the weight-related benefits vegetarians experience may be explained by non-dietary factors. These may include healthy lifestyle choices like exercising and other health-related decisions. That said, several studies have shown that vegan diets are quite effective for weight loss and weight management. Further studies report that folks who resort to vegan diets generally shed more pounds than those on calorie-restricted diets, regardless of the quantity they eat. Plus, vegans naturally consume fewer calories, which works towards speeding up weight loss.

Vegan diet, blood sugar and Type II Diabetes

You can keep your blood sugar and Type II Diabetes at bay by adopting a vegan diet. Studies have shown that vegans generally have higher insulin sensitivity, lower blood sugar levels, and over 75% less risk of developing Type II Diabetes than non-vegans. The ADA, NCEP, and AHA, report that vegan diets lower blood sugar levels in diabetics up to 2.5 times more than other diets. This can be explained, in part, by the high fiber intake, which blunts the blood sugar response. The weight loss effect associated with this diet further contributes to its ability to keep the blood sugar levels low.

Vegan diet and cardiovascular health

A vegan diet can help you have a healthy heart

Studies report that vegans have up to 75% lower risk of developing hypertension and 43% lower risk of dying from cardiovascular complications. Vegan diets are quite effective at reducing LDL, blood sugar, and total cholesterol than other diets.

Other health benefits associated with the vegan diet

Vegan diets have been linked with an array of multiple health benefits including the following:

- Cancer risks

The vegan diet can lower your risk of developing colon cancer by up to 15%

- Arthritis

Vegan diets are quite popular for managing the symptoms of arthritis such as swelling of the joints, pain, and morning stiffness

- Kidney function

Diabetics who give up meat for plant protein can lower their risk of poor kidney function tremendously

- Alzheimer's disease

Studies indicate that certain aspects of vegan diet can help reduce an individual's risk of developing Alzheimer's disease.

Foods to avoid while on a vegan diet

It should go without saying that animals products should not feature in the vegan diet. These include:

- Poultry and meat: lamb, beef, veal, organ meat, horse, wild meat, chicken, goose, turkey, duck, and quail.

- Fish and seafood: all kinds of fish, shrimp, anchovies, squid, calamari, scallops, crab, mussels, and lobster.

- Dairy: yogurt, milk, butter, cheese, ice cream, and cream

- Eggs

- Bee products: honey, royal jelly, pollen

- Animal based ingredients: casein, whey, lactose, gelatin, egg white albumen, isinglass, L-cysteine, cochineal or carmine, animal derived vitamins, and fish derived Omega-3 fatty acids

Foods to eat while on a vegan diet

Here are some of the plant-based foods you can substitute animal products for:

- Legumes: Foods such as lentils, beans, and peas are excellent sources of nutrients and beneficial plant compounds. You can increase nutrient absorption by sprouting, fermenting, and properly cooking them

- Tofu, tempeh and seitan: these foods are versatile protein-rich alternatives to beef, fish, and eggs

- Nuts and nut butters: unroasted and unblanched varieties are especially great sources of fiber, iron, zinc, magnesium, vitamin E, and selenium

- Seeds: especially chia, hemp, and flaxseeds contain good concentrations of proteins and are also rich in omega-3 fatty acids

- Calcium fortified plant milk and yogurts: these can help you achieve the recommended dietary calcium intake. You may also opt for varieties with vitamin B12 and D

- Algae: chlorella and spirulina are great protein sources. Other varieties are rich in iodine

- Nutritional yeast: this is a great option for increasing your protein intake and add an interesting cheesy to your diet. Always opt for vitamin B12-fortified varieties whenever you can

- Whole grains, cereals, and pseudo-cereals: these are great sources of fiber, complex carbs, B-vitamins, and several minerals. Teff, spelt, amaranth, and quinoa are especially rich in protein

- Fruits and vegetables: Both are excellent foods for increasing your nutrient intake. Leafy greens such as spinach, bok choy, kale, mustard greens, and watercress are specifically rich in calcium and iron

Risks and how to minimize them

Promoting a well-planned diet that limits processed foods while replacing them with nutrient-rich ones is important for pretty much everyone, not just vegans. That said, you risk suffering from a deficiency of certain nutrients when you poorly plan your vegan diet. In fact, research indicates that vegans are at a greater risk of having inadequate blood levels of vitamins B12 and D, iodine, long-chain omega-3s, calcium, zinc, and iron. Failing to get enough of these nutrients is worrisome for everyone; however, they pose a specific risk to infants as well as pregnant and breastfeeding mothers.

Your genetic composition, as well as the composition of your gut's bacteria, may also affect your ability to harness the nutrients you need from your vegan diet. One excellent way of minimizing the possibility of deficiency is to cut back on the amount of processed vegan foods in your meals and instead opt for nutrient-rich plant foods.

Fortified foods, especially those rich in vitamins B12 and D as well as calcium, should also feature prominently in your vegan diet. Furthermore, you should try fermenting, sprouting, and cooking your foods to enhance absorption of zinc and iron. Also, the use of cast iron pans and pots when cooking, avoiding coffee or tea with meals, and combining iron-rich foods with vitamin C sources can further boost the absorption of iron. Adding seaweed or iodized salt to your diet can also ensure that you realize the daily recommended iodine levels.

Finally, Omega-3 rich foods, especially those rich in alpha-linolenic acid (ALA), can help the body synthesize long-chain Omega-3s such as eicosapentaenoic acid (EPA) and docosahexaenoic acid (DHA). Foods rich in ALA include hemp, chia, flaxseeds, soybeans, and walnuts.

Some supplements you may want to consider while on vegan diet

Some vegans may encounter a challenge in getting enough of the fortified or nutrient-rich foods discussed above to meet their daily requirement. In that case, here are some supplements that you may find beneficial:

- Vitamin B12: Vitamin B12 present in cyanocobalamin is the most researched form and seems to work perfectly well for most people.

- Vitamin D: You may opt for D12 or vegan D3 forms

- DHA and EPA: these are processed from algae oil

- Iron: You may take this supplement in case there is a documented case of deficiency. Remember, ingesting high levels of iron can cause health complications and inhibit absorption of certain nutrients

- Iodine: you may take this as a supplement or add ½ teaspoon of iodized salt to your meals

- Calcium: this is best absorbed when taken in doses of 500 mg or less at a time. Avoid taking calcium with iron or zinc supplements as this may inhibit their absorption

- Zinc: you can get this in zinc gluconate or zinc citrate forms. Do not take together with calcium supplements

A one-week vegan sample menu

Monday

Breakfast

Start off with a vegan breakfast sandwich with lettuce, tofu, turmeric, tomato, and a plant-milk chai latte

Lunch

Spiralized zucchini with quinoa salad and peanut dressing

Dinner

Spinal dal and red lentil accompanied with wild rice

Tuesday

Breakfast

Overnight oats prepared with fruit, chia seeds and nuts, and fortified plant milk.

Lunch

Seitan sauerkraut sandwich

Dinner

Pasta accompanied with lentil Bolognese sauce and salad

Wednesday

Breakfast

A spinach and mango smoothie prepared with fortified plant milk and a flaxseed-banana-walnut muffin

Lunch

Baked tofu sandwich with a tomato salad

Dinner

Vegan chili on bed of amaranth

Thursday

Breakfast

Whole-grain toast accompanied by banana, hazelnut butter, and fortified plant yogurt

Lunch

Tofu noodle soup with veggies

Dinner

Jacket sweet potatoes with corn, lettuce, beans, guacamole, and cashews

Friday

Breakfast

Onion omelet and vegan chickpea and cappuccino prepared with fortified plant milk

Lunch

Vegan tacos with pineapple or mango salsa

Dinner

Tempeh stir-fry prepared with bok choy and broccoli

Saturday

Breakfast

Spinach with scrambled tofu wrap and a glass of fortified plant milk

Lunch

Spiced red lentil with tomato and kale soup, with hummus and whole-grain toast

Dinner

Miso soup, veggie sushi rolls, edamame and wakame salad

Sunday

Breakfast

Guacamole, chickpea pancakes, salsa, and a glass of fortified orange juice

Lunch

Tofu vegan quiche accompanied by a side of sautéed mustard greens

Dinner

Vegan spring rolls

Eating out as a vegan

Eating out as a vegan can be very challenging. The best way to reduce stress is to identify a vegan-friendly restaurant ahead of time. You can use websites like Vegguide and Happycow or applications like Vegman and VeganXpress to identify vegan friendly restaurants in your city.

When eating at a non-vegan friendly restaurant, always try to scan the menu beforehand to see the vegan options they might have for you. Sometimes, making that phone call ahead of time can allow the chef to prepare something especially for you. This allows you to arrive at the restaurant with confidence that you will have something more interesting than just a side salad.

While choosing a restaurant on the fly, try to find out about their vegan options as soon as you walk in, ideally before taking your seat.

Opt for ethnic restaurants when in doubt. They tend to have vegan-friendly dishes or can easily modify their dishes to be so. Thai, Mexican, Ethiopian, Middle-Eastern, and Indian restaurants too tend to be wonderful options when looking for vegan-friendly eateries.

Once in the restaurant, identify vegan friendly options on the menu by asking whether eggs or dairy have been removed to make the dishes vegan-friendly. You may also order several side dishes and vegan appetizers to make up your meal.

Some healthy vegan snacks

Snacks are an excellent way to stay energized and avoid hunger between your meals.

Here are some portable vegan options worth considering:

- Humus and vegetables
- Fresh fruit with a dollop of nut butter
- Roasted chickpeas
- Nutritional yeast sprinkled on popcorn
- Trail mix

- Nut and fruit bars
- Chia pudding
- Whole-wheat pita with guacamole and salsa
- Homemade muffins
- Edamame
- Cereal with plant milk
- Dried seaweed snacks
- Whole-grain crackers with cashew nut spread
- Cappuccino or plant-milk latte

Always try to enrich your vegan snack with fiber and protein sources to help keep hunger at bay.

Bottomline

People choose veganism for various reasons: environmental, ethical, and health reasons. When done right, this easy to follow diet can provide multiple health benefits including weight loss management. However, as with any diet, you will only realize these benefits if you are consistent and build your diet on nutrient-rich plant foods rather than heavily processed foods. Finally, a vegan who is unable to meet their daily nutrient requirement through diet alone should consider taking supplements.

Chapter 6: Low Carbohydrate Diet

A low-carb diet limits the intake of carbohydrates such as those found in starchy vegetables, grains, and fruits while emphasizing foods that are rich in fat and protein. Low-carb diet exists in different variations. Each low-carb diet variation restricts the types, and amount, of carbohydrates that you can eat.

Purpose of low carb diet

A low carbohydrate diet is generally perfect for weight loss. Some low carb diets may come with additional benefits beyond weight loss, such as managing the risk factors associated with metabolic syndrome and Type II Diabetes.

Why you might take to a low carb diet

You may follow a low carbohydrate diet due to one of the following reasons:

- When you want a diet that restricts the intake of certain carbohydrates to help you lose weight

- When you want to change your overall eating habit

- When you want to enjoy the types and amounts of foods featured in a low-carbohydrate diet

Like with any other weight loss diet plan, it is important that you check with your dietician or doctor before starting your low carb diet plan. This is specifically important if you have health conditions like diabetes and cardiovascular conditions.

Low carbohydrate diet details

As already indicated, this diet restricts the type and amount of carbs you should eat. Carbohydrates are a type of calorie-providing macronutrients present in most foods and beverages.

Carbohydrates can be simple or complex. Furthermore, they can be classified as simple natural (fructose in fruits and lactose in milk), simple refined (table sugar), complex refined (white floor), and complex natural (as found in grains like corn and beans).

Naturally occurring carbohydrates can be obtained from the following food groups:

- Vegetables
- Fruits
- Grains
- Milk
- Seeds
- Nuts
- Legumes like lentils, beans, and peas

Food processors may also add refined carbohydrates to their products in the forms of white flour or sugar. Examples of foods that contain refined carbohydrates include pasta and white breads, cake, cookies, candy, and sugar-sweetened drinks and sodas.

Your body utilizes carbohydrates as its primary source of fuel. The body breaks down complex carbohydrates like starches into simple sugars for absorption. The simple sugars are then absorbed into the blood stream where they are referred to as blood sugar "glucose". Generally, natural complex carbohydrates are broken down more slowly and they have less effect on your blood sugar levels. These complex carbohydrates provide bulk and serve other physiological functions beyond fueling the body.

The rising blood sugar levels trigger the pancreas to secrete insulin. Insulin helps the body to absorb glucose. Some glucose is used by the body for energy, enabling the physiological process to occur, fueling all your activities, whether it is simple breathing or going out for an exercise. The extra glucose, however, is stored in the muscles, liver, and other cells for later use or is converted to fat and stored in the adipose tissue.

The idea behind low carbohydrate diet is that reduced carbohydrate intake lowers insulin levels, which prompts the body to burn stored fat for energy resulting in weight loss.

Typical foods in the low carb diet

Generally, a low carb diet focuses on proteins, including poultry, meat, eggs, and fish as well as some non-starchy vegetables. This diet generally limits or totally excludes most legumes, grains, breads, fruits, sweets, starchy vegetables, pasta, and sometimes seeds and nuts. Some low carb diets allow small portions of certain fruits, whole grains, and vegetables.

The typical low carb diet comes with a daily limit of 20 to 60 grams (0.7 to 2 ounces). These amounts of carbs provide 80 to 240 calories. Some low carb diets strictly restrict carbohydrates during the initial phase of the diet before gradually increasing the number and amount of permissible carbs.

On the contrary, the Dietary Guidelines for Americans recommend that carbs should make up 45 to 65 percent of your daily calorie sources. Thus, if you consume 2,000 calories per day, you are advised to eat between 900 and 1,300 calories per day of carbs.

The results

Weight loss

Some people can lose weight if they cut back on the number of calories they consume and increase their physical activity. For instance, if you want to lose 1 to 1.5 pounds, (about 0.5 to 0.7kg) in a week, you should consider reducing your daily calorie intake by 500 to 750 grams.

Studies have shown that low carb diets, especially extremely low carb diets, may result is greater short-term weight loss than low-fat diets. However, further studies have shown that the weight loss benefits of low carb diets are not very extensive in the long-run, say 12 to 24 months. A 2015 study found that a low carb, higher-protein diet may offer a slight advantage in terms of weight loss as well as loss of fat mass compared to the normal protein diet.

But, restricting carbs and calories may not be the only reason for the weight loss. Some studies have found that you can lose some extra weight because the extra fat and proteins keep you feeling fuller for longer, which ensures that you eat less.

Other health benefits of low carb diets

A low carb diet may help manage, or prevent, severe health complications like diabetes, metabolic syndrome, high blood pressure, as well as cardiovascular diseases. In fact, any weight loss diet can reduce or even contain the risk factors associated with diabetes and heart problems. Additionally, most weight loss diets, not just low carbohydrate diets, tend to improve blood cholesterol as well as blood sugar levels.

In some people, low carbohydrate diet may

improve high-density lipoprotein (HDL) cholesterol and triglyceride levels slightly more than moderate carbohydrate diets. Besides the amount of carbs you eat in a low-carb diet, this is also attributed to the quality of the other foods you eat. Lean proteins like poultry, fish, and legumes, healthy fats like monounsaturated and polyunsaturated fats, and unprocessed carbohydrates like legumes, whole grains, vegetables, low-fat dairy products, and fruits are generally healthier options.

According to the American Heart Association, the Obesity Society, the American College of Cardiology, there is not sufficient evidence to say whether most low-carbohydrate diets provide heart healthy benefits.

Risks

When you suddenly and drastically cut carbs, you may experience a range of negative effects, such as:

- Bad breath

- Headache
- Weakness
- Fatigue
- Muscle cramps
- Skin rashes
- Diarrhea or constipation

Additionally, some diets restrict carb intake so much that, in the long run, they can result in mineral or vitamin deficiencies, gastrointestinal disturbances, bone loss, as well as increasing the risk of various chronic diseases.

Because low carbohydrates may not provide all the essential nutrients, these diets are not recommended for weight loss and management for pre-teenagers and high schoolers. Their growing bodies require nutrients found in fruits, whole grains, and vegetables.

Severely restricting your carbohydrate intake to

less than 20 grams (0.7 ounces) per day can trigger a process called ketosis. This occurs when the body does not have enough glucose (sugar) to convert to energy, triggering the body to break down stored fat. This causes ketones to build up in the body. The side effects of ketosis may include headache, nausea, physical and mental fatigue, and bad breath.

There is no information of the possible long-term health risks of low carb diets because most studies have lasted no more than one year. Some diet and health experts report that eating large amounts of protein and fat from animal sources may increase your risk of heart disease as well as increasing your chances of developing some cancers.

If you are on a low-carb diet that is high in protein and fat, it is important that you opt for foods that are rich in healthy proteins and healthy unsaturated fats. Consider limiting your intake of foods that are rich in saturated and trans fats such as high-fat dairy products, meat, and pastries and processed crackers.

Low carb diet: what to drink

What low carb alcohols can you drink? Some common mistakes? This section will guide you on what you need to know about drinks and low carb diet.

First of all, consuming a lot of alcohol will slow your weight loss. Besides, it may also undermine your health gains especially when you are on low-carb diet. The body breaks down alcohol before anything else, and this tends to slow down fat (and weight) loss.

However, drinking in moderation should not be a big deal as long as it is low in carbs. Low carb options include champagne, wine, and pure spirits like vodka and whiskey. High carb drinks include beers and sugary cocktails.

Foods to maybe include in your low carb diet

If you are healthy, active, and do not need to lose weight, you do not have to worry about a few more carbs.

- Tubers – sweet potatoes, potatoes, and other tubers

- Unrefined grains – oats, brown rice, quinoa, and many more

- Legumes – like lentils, pinto beans, and black beans

You may also have the following in moderation

Wine – opt for dry wine with no added carbs or sugar

Dark chocolate – especially organic brands that are at least 70% cocoa. Dark chocolate is an antioxidant that provides multiple health benefits when eaten in moderation. However, do remember that dark chocolate and alcohol can hinder your weight loss progress if you drink or eat too much.

Beverages for the low carb diet

- Tea
- Coffee
- Sugar-free carbonated beverages like sparkling water

A simple one-week low carbohydrate menu

This is a simple one-week menu inspired by a low-carb diet plan. It provides no more than 50 grams of carbs per day. However, you may take more carbs if you are healthy and active.

Monday

Breakfast

Omelet with vegetables fried in coconut oil or butter

Lunch

Grass-fed yogurt, with almonds and blueberries

Dinner

Bun-less cheeseburger served with veggies and salsa sauce

Tuesday

Breakfast

Bacon with eggs

Lunch

Burgers (possibly leftover from last night) and veggies

Dinner

Salmon with vegetables and butter

Wednesday

Breakfast

Pan fried eggs and vegetables, fried in coconut oil and butter

Lunch

Shrimp salad with olive oil

Dinner

Grilled chicken served with vegetables

Thursday

Breakfast

Omelet with vegetables, fried in coconut oil or butter

Lunch

Smoothie with berries, coconut milk, protein powder and almonds

Dinner

Steak and various vegetables

Friday

Breakfast

Bacon and eggs

Lunch

Chicken salad served with olive oil

Dinner

Pork served with various veggies

Saturday

Breakfast

Omelet served with various vegetables

Lunch

Grass-fed yogurt with coconut flakes, berries, and walnuts

Dinner

Meatballs served with vegetables

Sunday

Breakfast

Bacon and eggs

Lunch

Smoothie with a dish of heavy cream, coconut milk, berries, and chocolate flavored protein powder

Dinner

Grilled chicken served with raw spinach

Include a lot of low-carb vegetables in your diet. If your goal is to keep your intake at 50 grams of carbohydrates per day, there is room for lots of vegetables and one fruit each day. Again, if you are lean, healthy, and active, you may include some tubers like sweet potatoes and potatoes as well as healthy grains in your diet.

Healthy, low carbohydrate snacks

There is no health reason to take more than three meals in a day. However, if you get hungry between your meals, here are easy-to-prepare yet healthy low carbohydrate snacks to get you filled up:

- Full-fat yogurt

- A piece of fruit

- Baby carrots
- One or two boiled eggs
- Some cheese and meat
- A handful of nuts
- Leftover from the previous night

Eating at restaurants

It is easy to make your meals low-carb friendly while eating out. Here are some options:

- Order fish or meat-based main dish
- Take plain water instead of sugary fruit juice or soda
- Order extra veggies instead of potatoes, bread, or rice

A simple low carbohydrate shopping list

The best rule is to shop at the store's perimeter where you are more likely to find whole foods.

You will make your diet much better than the standard Western diet when you focus on whole foods.

Grass-fed and organic foods are quite popular choices and are often deemed healthier; however, they are typically expensive.

Consider choosing processed options that still fit into your budget.

- Butter

- Coconut oil

- Meat (lamb, beef, chicken, pork, and bacon)

- Lard

- Cheese

- Fish (fatty fish like salmon is great)

- Sour cream

- Heavy cream

- Blueberries
- Yogurt (unsweetened but full fat)
- Olives
- Nuts
- Fresh veggies (peppers, greens, onions)
- Condiments (seal salt, garlic, pepper, mustard)
- Frozen veggies (carrots, broccoli, various mixes)

Avoid unhealthy temptations like chips, ice cream, candy, juices, sodas, cereals, and baking ingredients like sugar and flour.

Bottom line

Low carb diet, as the name alludes, restricts the intake of carbohydrates such as those present in processed and sugary foods like white bread and pasta. This diet is rich in fat, protein, and healthy vegetables. Studies show that this diet can help with one's weight loss and improved health.

Chapter 7: Weight Loss and Fasting

A phenomenon known as intermittent fasting has recently gained popularity as one of the most effective fitness and weight loss methodologies. Basically, it involves alternating cycles of eating and fasting.

Studies have linked fasting to improved metabolic health, weight loss, and protection against lifestyle diseases like diabetes, and various heart conditions.

So what is intermittent fasting?

This is an eating pattern where you cycle between periods of fasting and eating. It does not mention the foods you should eat but rather when you should eat them.

There are different intermittent fasting methods, all of which split the day or week into fasting periods and eating periods. Of course, most folks already "fast" while asleep. And intermittent fasting can be as simple as extending that fast by a few hours. You may do this by skipping your breakfast and having your first meal of the day at noon and your last meal no later than 8pm. Thus, you will be technically fasting for around 15-16 hours per day while restricting your eating to an 8-hour eating window. Commonly known as 16/8, this is one of the most popular forms of intermittent fasting.

Despite what people say, intermittent fasting is quite easy to practice. Most people report a better feeling and rejuvenation while on this fast. Hunger is never a big deal, although it can be a challenge while starting when your body is getting used to not getting nourished with food for extended hours.

No food is allowed while fasting. However, you may drink water, tea, coffee, and other non-caloric beverages. In fact, you are encouraged to take lots of water while fasting.

Some variations of intermittent fasting permit small quantities of low-calorie foods during the fasting hours. Additionally, you may take supplements while fasting as long as there are no calories on them.

So why fast?

Well, man has actually been fasting for thousands of years. At times, this is done out of necessity when there simply was nothing to eat. In other instances, man fasted for religious reasons. Religions like Christianity, Islam, and Buddhism advocate some form of fasting.

People also instinctively fast when sick

Clearly, fasting is quite natural, and the human body is well equipped to handle extended periods without food. All sorts of physiological processes change when you go without food for a while in order to allow your body to thrive during times of famine. A lot of these processes have to do with genes, hormones, and important cellular repair processes.

Fasting causes a reduction in blood sugar as well as insulin levels. It also triggers a drastic rise in human growth hormone. Most people take to intermittent fasting to lose weight since it is a very simple yet effective way of restricting calories while burning fat. Yet, other people fast for metabolic health benefits as this can help manage various health markers as well as risk factors.

Some studies have linked intermittent fasting to longevity. A study conducted on rodents showed that fasting can extend a lifespan as effectively as calorie restriction. Some studies also indicate that intermittent fasting can protect against diseases such as Type II Diabetes, heart disease, some forms of cancer, Alzheimer's disease, amongst other health complications. And yet, other people just love the convenience of intermittent fasting.

Intermittent fasting is a simple "life hack" that makes your life simple while improving your overall health and wellbeing at the same time.

The fewer meals you have to plan for, the simpler your life is bound to be, no doubt. And, skipping 3-4 meals during the day, with the preparation and cleaning that comes with them, also saves a lot of time.

Intermittent fasting as a powerful tool for your weight loss

Most people try intermittent fasting to lose weight.

By eating fewer meals, intermittent fasting should automatically result in reduced calorie intake. Additionally, intermittent fasting triggers a change in the body's hormone levels to facilitate weight loss. By lowering insulin while increasing the growth hormone levels, fasting stimulates the release of the fat burning hormone norepinephrine (noradrenaline). Due to these hormonal changes, fasting for a short period can increase your metabolic rate by 3.5-15%.

By eating less while burning more calories, intermittent fasting triggers weight loss by changing both sides of the calorie equation. However, it is important to understand that the main explanation for its success is that intermittent fasting lets you consume fewer calories overall. However, if you are binge eating during your meal times, you may not lose any weight at all.

Types of intermittent fasting

Intermittent fasting has gained popularity over the past few years with different methods/types emerging. Here are some of the most popular intermittent fasting methods:

- The 16/8 intermittent fasting – This involves fasting for up to 16 hours per day, only having two meals at noon and 8pm.

- Eat-stop-eat – For one or two days in a week, do not eat anything for up to 24 hours, i.e. from dinner on day one to dinner the next day

- The 5:2 diet – During two days of the

week, limit your calorie intake to 500-600 calories.

How to lose weight with intermittent fasting

There are many different ways to lose weight, and intermittent fasting is one of them. Short-term fasting helps you eat fewer calories, and also helps optimize the hormones that are responsible for weight regulation. As long as you do not make up for unconsumed calories by increasing your food portions during non-fasting periods, intermittent fasting should result in reduced calorie intake while helping your lose weight and body fat.

Intermittent fasting and your hormones

The body stores extra energy (calories) in the form of body fat. When you do not eat anything, the body effects several changes to make the stored energy accessible for physiological function. This has something to do with the changes in the activities within your nervous system, as well as changes in other crucial hormones.

Here are some of the changes that happen to your metabolism when you fast:

- Insulin – Your insulin level rises when you eat. As you fast, on the other hand, insulin levels decrease dramatically. Lower insulin levels speed up the fat burning process.

- Human growth hormone (HGH) – Your growth hormone levels may shoot up during the fasting period, sometimes increasing as much as 5 times. Grow hormone has been established to promote fat loss and muscle gain.

- Norepinephrine (noradrenaline) – Due to changes in the nervous system during a fast, the body releases hormone norepinephrine into the fat cells, breaking them down into free fatty acids that can be utilized for energy.

Interestingly, despite what supporters of 5-6 meals a day would want you to believe, short-term fasting may actually speed up fat burning, and consequent weight loss. Studies have shown that fasting for about 48 hours can boost your metabolism by 3.5-15%. However, it is important to note that fasting for longer periods can suppress metabolism.

Intermittent fasting can help you hold on to muscle when dieting

One of the side effects of dieting is that the body tends to burn muscles as well as fats. Interestingly, studies have shown that intermittent fasting may be beneficial for retaining your muscles while burning body fat. In another study, intermittent fasting was found to restrict calories resulting in equivalent weight loss, but with a much smaller reduction in muscle mass.

Succeeding with intermittent fasting

There are certain things you need to keep in mind if you want to lose weight with intermittent fasting. Here are some of them:

- Food quality – The foods you eat during your intermittent fasting is important. Try to eat whole foods, with single ingredient foods.

- Calories – Yes, calories still count. It works best when you eat "normally" during your eating periods. Do not eat so much as to compensate for the calories you missed while fasting.

- Consistency – Just as with any other weight loss approach, intermittent fasting will only work if you follow through with it for an extended period of time.

- Patience – Certainly, it will take your body time to adjust to an intermittent fasting protocol. Be consistent with your eating schedule for a better outcome.

Most intermittent fasting methods also recommend strength training. This is key if you want to burn body fat while keeping your muscles. At the beginning of intermittent fasting, you do not have to count calories. However, calorie counting can be a useful tool if your weight loss stagnates.

Six popular ways to do intermittent fasting

Intermittent training has gained tremendous popularity in recent years. It can help you lose weight, improve your metabolic health, and help you live longer. Given its popularity, different methods/types of intermittent fasting have been devised. While all of them can be effective for weight loss, the one that best fits your weight loss needs to basically depend on your health and weight loss goals.

Here are six popular ways to fast intermittently

1. The 16/8 intermittent fasting method

This intermittent fasting method involves fasting each day for 15-16 hours, while restricting your daily "eating window" to 8-10 hours. You can fit in 2-3 or more meals during this eating window. Also, known as the Leangains protocol, the 16/8 intermittent fasting was first made popular by fitness expert Martin Berkhan. The 16/8 intermittent fasting can be as simple as not eating anything after your dinner and skipping breakfast. For instance, if you have your dinner at 8pm, then have your next meal the following day at noon. This is technically 16 hours of fasting between your meals. Women are advised to fast for 14-15 hours because they do better with relatively shorter fasts. And if you are the type that gets hungry in the morning and like to take breakfast, then you will need to work hard to get used to skipping breakfast. You may drink water, tea, and other non-caloric beverages while fasting to reduce your hunger levels.

2. The 5:2 diet – fast for two days

This intermittent diet plan involves normal eating 5 days of the week before restricting your calories to 500-600 on two days of the week. Popularized by British doctor and journalist Michael Mosley, this diet is also referred to as Fast diet. During the two fasting days, women are advised to take 500 calories while men are advised to take no more than 600 calories. For instance, you may eat normally every day except Tuesday and Friday when you resort to two small meals (250-300 calories each day).

3. Eat-Stop-Eat – Doing a 24-hour fast once or twice per week

Popularized by Brad Pilon, this intermittent fast involves a 24-hour fast either once or twice per week depending on your health and weight loss goals. You can fast from dinner one day to the next day's dinner, amounting to a 24-hour fast. Example, after eating dinner at 7pm on Sunday, do not eat anything until dinner the following day. You may fast from lunch to lunch or breakfast to breakfast. The end result is pretty much the same. If you are doing this to lose weight, then you need to eat during your eating days. Meaning, eat the same portion of food as if you were never fasting.

4. Alternate-Day fasting – fasting every other day

This fasting means eating one day and fasting the next. It comes in different variations. Some versions allow uptake of up to 500 calories during the fasting days. Most studies link this version of intermittent fasting to several health benefits. However, this form of fasting is rather extreme and should be done under the strict supervision of your doctor. Additionally, this form of fasting is not advisable for nursing mothers or individuals with certain medical conditions.

5. The warrior diet – Fasting during the day, eating a large portion

during the night

Popularized by fitness expert Ori Hofmekler, the Warrior Diet involves eating small amounts of vegetables and fruits during the day and a huge meal at night. Basically, it champions "fasting" during the day and "feasting" at night within a 4-hour eating window. This diet is one the first popular "diets" to incorporate a form of intermittent fasting. Its food choices are similar to the Paleo diet – whole, unprocessed foods that are as close to nature as possible.

6. Spontaneous meal skipping – skipping your meals when convenient

You do not have to follow a structured intermittent fasting plan to realize its benefits. Another popular version of intermittent fasting is to simply skip your meals at random, say when you are too busy to cook and eat or when you are not feeling hungry. Remember, your body is adequately equipped to handle periods of famine, let alone skipping a meal or two. So if you really do not feel like eating, go ahead and skip a meal. Traveling somewhere and cannot find something healthy to eat? Try a short fast.

Skipping a meal or two when you do not feel like eating anything is basically intermittent fasting. Just be sure to compensate for skipped meals with healthy foods at other meals.

Chapter 8: Weight Loss and Exercise

A recent study on both men and women revealed that exercise alone does not help with weight loss. But, the findings also indicate that, to benefit, you have to exercise quite a bit. Theoretically, exercise should contribute substantially to your weight loss. It can help you burn calories fast. And if you do not replace the burnt calories, your body will achieve negative energy balance, burn stored fat for fuel, and shed pounds.

But life and metabolism are neither fair nor predictable, as multiple studies on exercise involving humans and animals have shown. In these studies, participants lost less weight than expected, given the energy they spend during exercise. These studies concluded that exercises did compensate for the calories they burnt while exercising, either by moving less the rest of the day or by eating more. While these compensations were unwitting, they were effective.

So how do you lose weight through exercise?

So you want to make sure every sweat helps you burn more? Well, here are five exercising rules for weight loss for your consideration.

Get FITT

When it comes to ensuring that your body does not get too comfortable with your workout, be sure to warm up to the FITT principle. This is an acronym for Frequency, Intensity, Time, and Type – the four factors that determine the exact stress you need to subject your body to while exercising. Making changes to any of these "surprises" challenges your body in a new way. Keep in mind that as long as you force your body to adapt to progressively challenging exercises, it is going to burn more calories with every exercise session. It is when the body gets used to the current exercises that things start to plateau. To achieve optimum results, it is advisable that you change two of these variables every four to six weeks.

And HIIT

This is an acronym for High Intensity Interval Training. In a 2013 study, 20 participants participating in HIIT recorded a loss of 20 calories per minute – about twice as much as they lost while on long runs. Additionally, HIIT workouts also come with the extra benefit of the "after burn" effect, which you will never get from a steady-state cardio workout. Thus, rather than burning 250 calories from your 30-minute HIIT session, you can burn up to 40% more throughout the next day or so as the body recovers. You may adapt this HIIT regime: Perform all-out for 30 seconds, have a 10-second rest, and repeat for five minutes. Rest for a minute, then repeat 4 times.

Prioritize healthy eating

If you do not pay attention to what you are eating, you can exercise every single day as hard as you possibly can and fail to lose a single pound if the calories you are spending are equal to or less than the calories you are eating. Besides, feeding on junk can make your workouts feel a lot more difficult, so even if you think you are pushing yourself to the max, you are probably not. And, below max workouts, as you probably know, burn fewer calories. Experts recommend limiting sugar in your diets and in their place eating healthy fats, lean protein, and whole carbohydrates from vegetables, fruits, and whole grains.

Pick up some weight

Want more muscle? Burn more calories. While a pound of fat only burns into two calories per day, a pound of muscle burns about six calories and takes a lot less room. According to a 2015 study conducted by Harvard School of Public Health, people who do strength training gain less belly fat than those who do cardio exercises.

Never forget to fuel

While everyone has a unique pre- and post-workout nutrition plan, a Sports Medicine publication shows that eating carbohydrates before starting your workout can improve your performance during HIIT and endurance workouts. And tougher exercises are known to burn more calories, both during and after exercises.

Cardiovascular exercises and weight loss

Generally speaking, your body need to burn more calories (energy output) than you eat (energy input) in order to lose weight. Cardio is just one form of exercise that can help contribute to your "energy output". And there are different types of cardio exercises such as jogging, walking, and sprinting. Depending on your weight loss goals, some forms of cardio exercises are best suited for this than others. For instance, if you want to burn fat and shed some pounds, you are better off trying out Low Intensity Steady State (LISS) cardio. This is because walking, it has been established, burns more fat per calorie in comparison to jogging or sprinting. Keeping up a consistent, steady effort helps raise the heart rate and improve the body's natural ability to utilize oxygen properly.

Simply put, you need oxygen to break down fat for energy. Thus, the lower the intensity of the workout, the more oxygen will be available for the body to break down fat. Jogging or sprinting takes up most oxygen thus depriving the body of the oxygen required to break down fat. The result, instead of breaking down fat for energy, the body opts for other sources of energy like carbs.

Ten best cardio exercises for weight loss

Here are ten types of cardio exercises to help you lose weight fast and get the desired results.

1. Elliptical

This equipment was originally designed to

minimize impact on hips and knee while still allowing for an excellent workout. Because its impact is relatively low, the calorie burning effect is not as great as other cardio exercise equipment like Stairmasters and treadmills. However, the elliptical machine can be an excellent way of burning calories without wearing your joints out. While the average 190-pound adult may only burn 500-600 calories per hour, if they are going at an above moderate rate, you can get even more out of your workout by adjusting the intensity, speed, and resistance.

Burning fat on an elliptical

Consider adding a high incline to activate extra leg muscles, especially your glutes. To increase the resistance, lower the incline so you can have a cross-country skiing feel to your workout that really works your quads. As with the stepmill, do not hold onto the handles or rails too lightly as this will reduce your efforts and lead to wrist or shoulder pain.

2. Running at a moderate pace

Running at a steady, yet moderate pace is an excellent way of burning fat and calories. However, it is not a prudent route for those looking to build or maintain muscles. According to experts, a 190-pound adult can burn 950 calories per hour while running at 8.5 miles per minute. This would be a wonderful, long run to do once per week to keep your aerobic capacity at its optimum. So get your running shoes on and shed some pounds while keeping your heart healthy.

How to burn fat while running

Experts recommend setting the incline at 2-3% if you are running on a treadmill to simulate outdoor running. This will help you burn more calories while being easy on your knees. If you find running boring, join a local running club or try different routes in your neighborhood. You are likely to cover more miles when running with a partner than when running alone.

3. Stair climbing

Stair climbing offers another excellent way to burn fat and calories. However, a 180 pound adult can only burn 500-600 calories at a moderate pace. Since it involves higher leg lift, climbing uses significantly more muscles than walking. This strengthens your limbs in a functional way. The only drawback is stair climbing puts a lot of weight and pressure on the joints, so it can be a bad idea for folks with bad knees.

The best way to burn fat while stair climbing

Try to incorporate 90% or more effort in stair climbing for 30 seconds with a one to two-minute recovery period. Doing 15-20 rounds will certainly spice up your workout while ensuring that you burn as many calories as possible.

4. Rope jumping

There is a reason why jump rope is part of a professional boxer's workout regime: it is easy to do, cheap, increases foot speed, and yes it burns a ton of calories. Think of your favorite fighter (whether wrestler or boxer), they all jump rope. Besides enhancing coordination, shoulder strength, and footwork, rope jumping also stimulates sprinting, allowing you to burn as much as 500 calories in under 45 seconds!

How to burn with rope jumping

While not many people can jump rope for half-an-hour, it is best to start off with intervals of slow and fast jumps. Start by jumping as much as you can in one minute before resting for 30 seconds. Repeat until you are through with your target. If you travel a lot, be sure to have your jump rope in your suitcase for a great workout without having to leave the comfort of your hotel room.

5. Kettlebells

While a kettlebell exercise is not exclusively a cardio-only workout, its calorie-burning power is too strong to overlook. A kettlebell exercise brings the best of both worlds: cardio and strength training. Additionally, a recent study puts kettlebell's calorie-burning effects at around 20 calories per workout minute. This total accounts for both the aerobic calorie expenditure as well as the anaerobic calorie burnt. Very few cardio exercises result in muscle buildup, and this is one of the exceptions. A good kettlebell workout can help you burn around 400-600 calories in 30 minutes.

The best way to burn calories with kettlebell exercise

If you can do 40-50 reps of a particular move, chances are your kettlebell is not heavy enough. Point is, neither go too light nor too heavy. The best way to lose weight with kettlebell exercise is to find one that lets you do a round for 30-40 seconds before resting for 20 seconds. You may set your timer for 30 minutes to see how many rounds you can go.

6. Cycling

While stationary bikes are a mainstay at most gyms, there is a reason why most folks never queue in line to use them: you have to be ready to go at an intense rate! So no pedaling with one eye on your social media account. The average 180-pound adult can burn as much as 1,150 calories per hour during vigorous indoor cycling. A moderate ride, on the other hand, can burn half that amount, about 675 calories, in an hour.

How to burn calories cycling

Doing intervals on a stationary bike is an excellent way to maximize your calorie burn in the shortest time possible. Start out by keeping the intensity high on the intervals for a couple of minutes before slowing down for a minute or so. Repeat this for as long as you can.

7. Swimming

Swimming is a complete body workout that starts the moment you hop into water. You are basically fighting gravity, so your muscles are doing their best to keep you afloat without a break until you get out of the water. Thus, with just one minute of swimming, you will have burnt 14 calories! Keep in mind that the type of stroke makes a difference. You will burn more calories with a butterfly stroke than a breast stroke, so be sure to incorporate different strokes while swimming.

How to burn calories while swimming

The easiest way to burn fat while swimming is to simply tread water. You may do a few laps before having a water-treading interval. If you can swim at a high level then take advantage of it and swim as fast as you can for as long as you possibly can. If you are not such a strong swimmer, then swim in intervals. Swim as fast as you can through the pool before swimming back the same distance at a slower pace. Consider alternating these patterns for the duration of your swimming exercise.

8. Rowing

Take a look at any collegiate rower's body and the chances are their v-cut frame will leave you envious. Rowing makes it into the list of top fat burning exercises because it is an excellent way of incorporating the upper and lower body in a low-stress manner on the joints. It can also help you work out the posterior area. At a moderate pace, a 180 pound adult can burn 800 calories after rowing for an hour.

The best way to burn fat rowing

Always keep your chest up and engage your entire body while rowing. Also, do not leave all the work to your hands – try using your legs too to get going. Here is an example of a rowing workout session: Row 250 meters as fast as you can in 20 minutes. Take a one-minute rest and repeat the row.

9. High intensity interval training

High intensity interval training (HIIT) provides a well-rounded exercise while burning lots of fat and calories. The outcome of a HIIT workout can vary greatly, from 500 calories per hour to over 1500 calories per exercise hour for a 180 pound adult. HIIT exercises are excellent because of the intensity of each workout as well as their reps and variations. Pair any body-weight movement with a weighted movement and some cardio workout for an excellent fat burning exercise.

How to burn calories with HIIT

Get HIIT, Tabata, high impact aerobic, and vigorous interval classes using your local gym's weights. It is important that you keep rest periods to a minimum in order to maximize your efforts and shed as much weight as you can.

10. Sprinting

Sprinting outdoors, on a treadmill, or on the stairs is an excellent way to burn the most calories in the shortest time possible. You do not need any equipment and you can sprint just about anywhere. While a steady-state jog can help you burn a lot of fat, increasing your speed and intensity will definitely pay off in a great way.

How to sprint away from calories

If you are running outdoors, try out a sprinting lap before doing a jogging lap. Repeat this for as long as you can. If you are sprinting on a treadmill, try an all-out sprint for 20-30 seconds before slowing the belt down for a one-minute jog before repeating. If you are jogging on the stairs, run up the stairs as fast as you can, then jog your way down.

Helpful tips for cardio exercises

If you are trying to lose weight, you know how it goes. You have to work out and watch what you eat. Simple. Specifically, you have to do both strength and cardio exercises to get the most out of your workout. In fact, cardio exercise is one of the most important arsenals you need for your weight loss journey. However, figuring out how much cardio you need, how hard you should work, and the right cardio exercises for your weight loss and fitness goals can be quite confusing. While this may be confusing, the upshot is to have a variety of choices so you do not have to do the same exercises at the same intensity day after day. In fact, you stand a chance of getting better results when you mix up your exercises. Working out at different intensities and combining your exercises will keep both your body and mind from getting bored.

If you are a beginner, you do not have to work so hard at your workouts from the onset. In fact, you should take your time, figure out the activities you enjoy, and consistently build endurance. The key is knowing what works for you.

How cardio can help you lose weight

By now, you probably know that weight loss only happens when you create a calorie deficit by burning more calories than you eat. While some folks prefer cutting calories through diet, it works better when you combine things – strength and cardio training, and health, low-calorie diet. All these are important, but cardio is a crucial component for the following reasons:

- You get to burn more calories during a single workout session – Getting your pulse to get to your desired heart rate zone means that your blood is pumping, you are breathing hard, and you are sweating. This is the calorie burning zone, and it should be your target if you really want to lose weight with cardio. And the harder and longer you work out, the more calories you will burn. For instance, a 180-pound adult can seamlessly burn 200 calories or more during a brisk 30-minute jog.

- You can easily adjust the intensity to increase your calorie burn – With cardio workout, it is easy to increase your calorie burn by regulating the intensity: jumping higher, going faster, climbing hills, or trying out new workouts that your body is not used to.

- It contributes to your overall calorie deficit – Burning fat through exercise means you do not have to eliminate as many calories from your diet. That is as long as you do not compensate for the exercise by eating more food after your workout, which may happen to some people.

- You can do cardio most days of the week – When lifting weights, your muscles require rest in order to recover and grow stronger. You can do cardio exercises most days of the week without worrying about picking up an injury or overtraining, depending on how you set up your workout regime.

The best cardio exercises

So you know you need cardio for weight loss, but which exercises are ideal and how much of them do you need to lose weight?

Well, the truth is, there really is no such thing as the BEST cardio exercise for weight loss. Rather, the best activity is the one you will consistently do and reach your weight loss goals. Never do anything that leaves you feeling miserable.

Having said that, some cardio exercises offer more intensity than others:

- Impact workouts – Workouts that involve some impact like walking or jogging will certainly boost your heart rate faster than non-impact exercises like cycling and swimming

- High impact activities – High impact workouts like running will certainly burn more calories than low impact ones like walking. Sometimes, you never quite have to do an entire exercise with high impact moves. You can simply identify a few and incorporate them into your workout plan and you will burn more calories

- Whole body activities – When you are working out both your upper and lower body, as in cross-country skiing, you are more likely to get your heart rate going and burn more fat. You can also achieve this by doing compounded strength exercises. When done right, you will not only get great cardio benefits but also build strength and endurance

This does not mean that you should ignore low impact workouts. Both types of exercises present great opportunities to burn calories, and doing both will give you a well-rounded workout regime.

In fact, it is in your best interest to combine both workouts as some exercises are challenging while others allow you to recover while exercising. It is important that you spend as much time as possible outside your comfort zone. You can accomplish this with intensive training or exercising hard for a short time before getting into the recovery phase. This is a wonderful way of burning calories while building your endurance.

To figure out how many calories you can burn with cardio exercises, take a look at this list of common exercises and the number of calories they can help you burn in 30 minutes:

- Stationary bike – 238 calories
- Step aerobics – 340 calories
- Walking at 5 mph – 175 calories
- Swimming – 270 calories
- Running at 5 mph – 270 calories
- Mowing your lawn – 200 calories

As you can see, everything from a simple walk to mowing the lawn can burn a significant number of calories, which underpins the importance of cardio for weight loss. You can turn almost any physical activity into a cardio workout if you work hard enough at it.

So how much cardio do you need?

There is no clear cut answer to how much cardio

you need to lose weight. However, there are guidelines that can give you a place to start, after which you can have a clearer idea of what your body can handle. The American Heart Association and the American College of Sports Medicine recommend about 20 to 40 minutes of moderate to vigorous intensity workout most days of the week. However, the truth of the matter is, the amount of cardio you need varies from person to person and is subject to factors such as:

- Your daily average calorie intake
- How you exercise
- Your age, gender, and metabolism
- Your body fat to weight ratio
- Your fitness level
- Your workout schedule

That said, here are tips for setting up an effective cardio workout regime:

Setting up a cardio workout program for a beginner

- If you are just getting started, pick an activity that feels good to you. You are better off starting with walking because you can do it anywhere and almost every day. Besides, you can set your pace when walking up or down hills. You can also add walking poles to increase the intensity.

- Start off with 3-4 days of activity, exercising at a moderate intensity. This is slightly out of your comfort zone.

- Exercise for as long as you can, pushing for 20 or more minutes per session.

- Add time to each week's exercise to work your way to 45 mins per session.

- As you build strength, try out interval training once per week to boost your endurance and burn more calories.

- Work your way up to 5-6 days of cardio and try different variations.

The bottom line is cardio can help you burn fat and lose weight. It is most effective when combined with strength training and a healthy, low-calorie diet.

Weight lifting and weight loss

Weight training is the new fad, make no mistake. Men and women across the country are hitting the gym to sack off the stereotypes – and if you are setting yourself up for weight loss, you might want to consider joining a weight lifting program.

Once upon a time, there was a fear that weight lifting would "bulk" one up. But more and more folks are realizing that lifting lots of weight can actually help shift the kilos.

If weight loss is your goal, the quickest way to shed some pounds would be by jogging mindlessly for an hour at the park or on the treadmill or taking a beasting in a spin –

although both are wonderful forms of workout and are great fun. However, lifting weights is an excellent way of burning lots of calories.

However, it is important to understand that it is not during the weight lifting activity that weight loss happens. This happens during the after-burn. While jogging burns lots of calories, keep in mind that everything stops when you stop. Weight lifting, on the other hand, can help you burn calories for up to 72 hours afterwards.

But calorie burn is not the only benefit that comes with weight lifting. Besides making you fitter and stronger, weight lifting also leaves a positive impact on your bone density while reducing your chances of developing osteoporosis. Some studies also claim that weight lifting can reduce your risk of developing cardiovascular disease as well as Type II Diabetes.

Ready to take to on weight lifting to shift the numbers on the scales? Well, here are five surefire ways to get the results you are looking for in the most efficient way.

1. Invest in your safety

Look, personal training = $$$, but a little bit of tuition can go a long way in reducing your chance of hurting yourself, and that certainly, makes the upfront cost worth it. At the very least, experts recommend having someone around to show you basic moves and how to use the weight equipment safely. It is important that you get the technique right – at best, you may never gain much, at worst you could end up hurting yourself! If you are not available for a one-on-one sesh, consider joining an instruction class.

2. Lift heavy

Bicep curling 1kg a few times is, obviously, not going to do anything for you – really! You need to be doing what professional weight lifters call "lifting to failure" – if you get to your third or fourth set of 10 reps. You need to be making only 9 or 10 max. If you are finding it easy, it is definitely a sign that you need to pick up a much heavier weight. After all, nobody said it was going to be easy.

3. Use your time wisely

Thanks to modern life, most people do not have the time to spend at the gym every day. However, that is not necessary when it comes to weight training. You just need to identify the moves that will take you where you want to be with your weight loss effort. Deadlifts, squats, and pull ups are excellent for working on big muscle groups.

4. Eat enough protein

Protein is important for building muscle. As such, eating a diet that is rich in fish, lean meats, eggs, nuts, eggs, and pulses should be an essential part of your training plan. Aim for 2-3 portions of healthy proteins per day. Good quality protein will keep you fuller for longer, you are less likely to undermine your progress with a 4pm sugar fix – after all, as old age approaches, you will not succeed in out-training a bad diet.

5. Be in calorie deficit

Still, the easiest and quickest way to lose weight is to burn more than you eat. It used to be believed that you could not build muscle in a calorie deficit. However, studies show that this is not the case. It is possible to reduce your calorie intake and report wonderful gains in calorie-consuming muscle at the same time. According to the NHS, an adult female can lose weight at a steady rate of 1400 calories per day. However, this is subject to your starting weight, activity levels, and height, amongst other factors. It is important that you talk to your doctor if you are not sure what is right for you.

The best weight lifting exercises for weight loss

By now, you clearly know the basic formula to drop pounds: eat less and move more. And, obviously, there are ways you can optimize this formula.

As far as moving goes, there are two types of

workouts that will help you burn more calories than the "traditional" exercises. Endurance workouts – think a long-distance swimmer or a marathoner – burn lots of calories because it takes a lot of energy to exercise for over two hours. The other type of workout is a little easier on your schedule: brief, high-intensive bouts that burn calories both during as well as after the workout, thanks to the metabolism-boosting effect called the "afterburn".

Here are 10 calorie burning workouts that can help you trim down your waist size.

Warming up

Do 30 yards or 20-30 seconds of each of the following workouts:

- Skips (stationary or traveling)
- Frankenstein kicks/walks
- Butt-kicks (stationary or traveling)
- Walkout pushups

- Walking (or alternating) lunges
- Walking (or stationary) knee hugs

Basic bodyweight workout

Unable to go to the gym? No problem. Take up these bodyweight exercises and burn calories anywhere, anytime. Do each workout for a minute each four times, with a 30 second rest, before repeating, for 30 minutes.

Do these exercises 3-4 times. Take a minute for each circuit.

- Jumping jacks
- Pushups
- V-sit ups
- Forward-backward lunges (30 seconds of each leg)
- Burpees
- Side stepping squats (30 seconds each leg)

- Mountain climbers

Beast mode bodyweight exercises

This exercise raises your body temperature while increasing your metabolism. Attempt the main circuit 2-3 times, taking as little rest as possible. Finish up with the cardio burnout.

Do each circuit for 30 seconds

- Windshield wipers
- Squats
- Isometric squats
- Reverse lunges (both left and right)
- Sumo squat jumps
- Plunk tricep get-ups (both left and right hands)
- Wide hand push-ups
- Side plank rotation with reach

- Renegade rows with pushups between

Then do 30 seconds of the following:

- Skater jumps
- Speed squats
- Burpees
- Quick feet
- High knee stationary sprint
- Speed jumping jacks

Classic gym circuit

If you do not have much time, and are happy with a simple workout, consider this effective circuit. Attempt the whole workout 3-5 times through, with as minimal rest as possible between the exercise sets. Use a heavy weight to finish the last reps.

Attempt the following workouts 4-5 times:

- 15 dumbbell squats with shoulder press

- 20 leg presses
- 15 hamstring curls
- 25 crunches
- 15 bench presses
- 10 tricep pressdowns
- 25 cable rows
- 10 dumbbell bicep curls

Tabata

The epitome of high intensity, tabata, will get you alternating 20 seconds of extreme effort with 10 seconds of rest repeated for four minutes. The beauty of tabata exercise is that you can perform short but intense workouts with your own body weight from the comfort of your home. This workout raises your heart rate, increase blood circulation, builds muscle, and improves your fitness level. The following tabata exercises will have you alternating two workouts while targeting the same muscle group and moving from one to the next provides the perfect kick-butt exercise in just 24 minutes.

- Lower body tabata #1 (repeat the circuit 4 times)

    - 20 seconds of speed squats followed by 10 seconds of rest
    - 20 seconds of isometric squat hold followed by 10 seconds of rest

- Lower body tabata #2 (repeat the circuit four times)

    - 20 seconds of walking lunges followed by 10 seconds of rest
    - 20 seconds of squat jumps followed by 10 seconds of rest

- Upper body tabata #1

    - 20 seconds of dumbbell bentover rows followed by 10 seconds of rest
    - 20 seconds of dumbbell chest press followed by 10 seconds of rest

- Upper body tabata #2 (repeat the circuit four times)
    - 20 seconds of dumbbell bicep curls followed by 10 seconds of rest
    - 20 seconds of dumbbell tricep kickbacks followed by 10 seconds of rest
- Cardio tabata (repeat the circuit four times)
    - 20 seconds of skater jumps followed by 10 seconds of rest
    - 20 seconds of frog jumps followed by 10 seconds of rest
- Tabata abs (repeat the circuit four times)
    - 20 seconds of bicycle crunches followed by 10 seconds of rest
    - 20 seconds of supermans followed by 10 seconds of rest

Battle ropes

If you have never made battle ropes part of your workout regime, you will soon find out why they are excellent for burning calories. Repeat this exercise four times for an excellent 20 minute kick-ass workout.

- A minute of rope alternating arm waves followed by 30 seconds of pushups

- A minute of rope double-arm slam jumping waves followed by 20 seconds of bicycle crunches

- A minute of rope outside crunches followed by 30 seconds of mountain climber

- Rest for 30 seconds and repeat

Killer kettlebells

Exercising with kettlebells is beneficial because it improves your body composition, generates body power, builds strength, and, of course, burns calories. Due to their weight distribution, kettlebells compel your muscles to counterbalance, thus improving your balance and stability as well. Perform these workouts unilaterally, meaning with one arm at a time, to further engage your core. Transition from one move to the next, then rest for about 30 seconds before repeating the entire workout 2-3 more times.

Perform ten reps each arm or leg. Do the complete group of workouts as a circuit, totaling to 3 circuits.

- Single arm swings
- Single arm bentover rows
- Squat to single arm overhead press
- Single-leg Russian deadlifts
- 45-60 second rest

TRX training

TRX exercises not only improve the body's total strength to burn more calories throughout the day, but also increases your heart rate and improves the body's composition. Additionally, this workout engages more of your core muscles. And with all of your core muscles being worked out, your entire body will be conditioned to result in tight lower abs at the same time.

Perform each of the following TRX exercises for 30 seconds:

Set one (repeat 3 times)

- TRX pushups
- TRX squat jumps
- TR pullups

Set 2 (repeat 3 times)

- TRX tricep extensions
- TRX reverse lunge to knee up (both sides)

- TRX bicep curls

Set 3 (repeat 3 times)

- TRX pike ups
- TRX hamstring curls

Set 4 (repeat 3 times)

- Side oblique crunches (both sides)

Fiery 50

Getting down to do abs, combo sprinting, and jump up as high as you can for the burpees can certainly help you burn through a lot of calories. Repeat the following workout 5-10 times without rest between the exercises with only 60 seconds of rest between rounds.

- 50 yard sprint
- 50 sit ups
- 50 yard reverse sprint (running backwards)

- 50 reverse sit ups

- 10 burpees

Metabolic strength

A metabolic exercise increases your strength and stamina, increases your metabolism, burns fat, and boosts energy levels and weight loss. But, the key to burning more calories with this workout is not in scrimping on the load and moving from one workout to the next without taking a break.

Do each exercise for 45 seconds with a heavy enough weight. You may use the same weight for the first four exercises and a lighter one for the last three. Rest 2-3 minutes at the end of each circuit before repeating everything 4 more times.

Repeat the circuit 2-3 times

- Barbell push press

- Barbell squat

- Barbell front squat

- Pushups
- Barbell bent over row
- Barbell skull crushers
- Barbell walking lunges
- Barbell standing bicep curls

Try-a-Tri

Do not overlook those long duration workouts. Hit the tracks, trails, and water for a long-duration fat burning workout. As a bonus, this could be your bonus prep for a triathlon. Take the shortest possible breaks to transition from one activity to the next.

- Swim for a quarter a mile (in the pool, lake, or ocean)
- Bike for 10 miles
- Run for 3 miles

High Intensity Interval Training

(HIIT) for Weight Loss

High intensity interval training involves combining bursts of workouts with short resting periods or light work (like walking or jogging – often referred to as active recovery. During the intervals, your heart rate should be at 80% of your maximum.

So just how intense is intense? Well, one way to assess the intensity of an exercise is to think about whether you could have a chat with a friend while working out. During HIIT, you should be exercising hard enough that you can barely hold a conversation.

Obviously, intensity is key, which means that you will really need to work

HIIT is basically a series of cardio workouts arranged as brief bursts of very tough exercises. The whole point of a high intensity exercise is to kick up your cardio's intensity. To qualify as a HIIT, you will need to push yourself to the maximum during each set. That explains why they have to be short – ranging from 30 to 90 seconds. Typically, HIIT is the opposite of opting for a long jog where you budget your energy in order to sustain the jog for longer.

Compared to other cardio exercises, HIIT can be an excellent way to lose weight. Additionally, HIIT workouts that involve bodyweight such as push-ups, or added weight such as medicine balls, kettlebells, or dumbbells will certainly tone your muscles while improving your heart rate and blood circulation. This workout is effective on multiple fronts: it improves endurance, complements strength development, and helps you burn calories.

Taking a break to rest is an important component of HIIT

Most people overlook the importance of rest while on high intensity interval training. But here is the point: rest periods between each session are an important part of the exercise. You are not getting it right if you are not taking time to recover.

Recovering before the next workout session is important, and here is why: forcing the body to repeatedly adjust between two different conditions provides excellent cardio conditioning. When your body works to adapt from the anaerobic (high-intensity) session to an aerobic recovery period during HIIT, this workload results in high calorie expenditure, which translates into weight loss. You need rest periods to prepare your body and enable it to perform at its maximum during the workout session.

How to ensure that you are getting HIIT right

HIIT rules are simple: exercise really hard, rest, then repeat! If you are enrolled in a fitness class or are working with a trainer, they will time your sets and rest periods and provide professional guidance as you work out. But you really do not need a world class gym, a workout plan, or even any equipment to reap big benefits with HIIT. Rather, all you need is activities that shoots your heart rate up, and then incorporate the HIIT approach to them.

A great starting point for beginners is with a 1:2 ratio of exercise to rest. Ideally, opt for all out on your chosen exercise for, say, 30, 45, or 60 seconds, rest for twice as long, then repeat the next set. You can transition to a 1:1 ratio as you get used to the workout. You can use assault bike, sprint, or run up the stairs. It is all HIIT as long as there is intensity.

A typical HIIT session should last for about 20-45 minutes of exercise and rest.

HIIT is a wonderful weight losing exercise, you should not be doing it alone.

As you probably already know, too much is definitely not a good thing. An overkill will most likely prevent you from optimizing your true capacity during your HIIT sessions. Therefore, do not schedule your HIIT session every day of the week. Rather, try HIIT three times per week with another 2 days dedicated to moderate cardio exercises.

It is important to understand that HIIT is not for everyone. Therefore, if you are training for a special goal or race, it is important that you follow an appropriate training regime – and HIIT may not be part of that regime. Due to the intensity level involved, always check with your doctor before embarking on a HIIT workout, as with any other exercise.

Finally, if you are doing HIIT for weight loss, the old adage that you cannot out-train a bad diet still holds, even if your workouts are super intensive. HIIT should not be an excuse to neglect your diet. So ensure that you keep it healthy, calculate your daily calorie needs, and plan your energy needs around your workout. You will only reap the desired results when you incorporate effective HIIT exercises into your workout regime and stay conscious of what you are eating.

Getting started with HIIT

Ready to jump right into your HIIT workout? Well, the truth is you can accomplish much with bodyweight workouts, an interval timer, and (most important) a positive attitude – you will need this when your legs start feeling like jelly!

You can start out by alternating sets of boxing jabs with jumping hacks and sumo squats to get your heart rate up and muscles burning.

Want a low-impact version to protect your knees? You can try out a 10-minute workout that combines runner's lunges, squat kicks, and plank twists, for a super-powered sweat-fest.

Always pay attention to your body when exercising at high intensity, and remember to have water breaks during and after your workouts to stay dehydrated.

It is easy to overdo things during your HIIT exercise, so ensure that you train with a group or a certified personal trainer. This will help you master your moves and get the most out of your exercises – all while keeping injuries off.

Benefits of HIIT

Besides providing the benefits that come with short-term exercises, HIIT also provides some unique health benefits.

1. HIIT can help you burn lots of calories in a short time

Yes, you can shred calories quickly using HIIT exercises

A recent study found that a 30 minute HIIT training that includes weight lifting, biking, and running, can burn 25-30% more calories than other forms of exercises. This is because HIIT lets you burn about the same amount of fats but spend less time working out.

2. Your metabolic rates remain high for hours after exercise

One of the ways HIIT helps you burn calories

actually comes after you are through with the exercise. Multiple studies have reported HIIT's remarkable ability to keep your metabolic rate high for hours after your workouts. Other studies have found out that HIIT can increase your metabolism after exercise than other workout forms like weight training and jogging. This workout shifts the body's metabolism toward burning existing fat rather than using the carbs you have eaten. Finally, another study revealed that a 2-minute HIIT workout that incorporates sprinting increased metabolism over 24 hours as much as 30 minutes of jogging.

3. HIIT can help you burn fat

Studies show that HIIT can help you burn fat and lose weight. In addition, a study found that folks performing HIIT three times per week for 20 minutes per session lost 2kg, 4.4 pounds, of body fat after 12 weeks of exercise – without making changes to their diet. And more important was the 17% reduction in visceral fat, the disease causing fat that is responsible for promoting most lifestyle conditions.

Several studies confirm that, despite its low time commitment, HIIT exercise can greatly reduce body fat. However, like other workout forms, HIIT can be extremely effective for fat loss in overweight or obese people.

4. HIIT can help you build muscle

Besides weight loss, HIIT can help you build up muscle. However, a gain in muscle mass happens in the muscles in most use, often the trunk and leg muscles. It is important to understand that an increase in muscle mass is more likely to occur in less active individuals. Studies in active individuals have not shown high muscle build up after HIIT exercises. Weight training remains the ultimate form of exercise for those seeking to build up muscle, with high-intensity intervals supporting small amounts of muscle growth.

5. HIIT can help improve oxygen circulation and consumption

Oxygen consumption refers to the muscles' ability to take up oxygen from the blood, and high intensity training is basically used to improve an individual's oxygen consumption. Basically, this consists of extended sessions of continuous cycling or running at a steady rate. However, it has been proven that HIIT can product similar benefits in a shorter amount of time. One study reported that five weeks of HIIT workouts performed 4 days per week for per 20 minute session can improve oxygen consumption by up to 10%. This is almost identical to the improvement in oxygen consumption in people who cycle for 40 minutes per day, 4 days per week. Yet, another study indicated that eight weeks of workouts on a stationary bike using HIIT or traditional exercise increased oxygen consumption by 25%. Additional studies support HIIT's improved oxygen consumption ability.

6. HIIT can reduce heart rate and blood pressure

Several studies indicate that HIIT exercises can

help reduce heart rate and blood pressure in obese and overweight individuals, who often grapple with high blood pressure. In one study, it was reported that 8 weeks of HIIT on a stationary bike reduced blood pressure the same way traditional continuous endurance training did in adults with high blood pressure. During this study, HIIT training group exercised 20 times per day, 3 times per week, while endurance training individuals exercised 30 minutes per day, four days per week. Other studies established that HIIT may even lower blood pressure more than the often recommended moderate-intensity exercises. However, it is important to mention that high-intensity workouts do not typically change blood pressure in normal weight folks with normal blood pressure.

7. You can reduce blood sugar level with HIIT

You can lower your blood sugar level with less than 12 weeks of consistent HIIT training.

According to multiple studies, HIIT not only reduces blood sugar but also improves an individual's insulin resistance more than traditional continuous workouts. Based on this finding, it is safe to report that high-intensity exercise can be particularly beneficial for folks at the risk of Type II Diabetes. In fact, experiments on individuals with Type II Diabetes have proven the effectiveness of HIIT for improving blood sugar. Finally, a study on healthy individuals indicate that HIIT can help improve insulin resistance even more than the traditional continuous exercises.

Top 10 HIIT workouts for weight loss

Ready to burn calories with HIIT exercises? Well, here are the best HIIT exercises that can help you burn fat, build muscles and stamina, and lose weight. And the beautiful thing is you can do these exercises at home.

1. HIIT for beginners

High intensity interval training is, without doubt, difficult for any beginner. However, with consistency, your fitness will adjust and you will be able to do your HIIT exercises with much ease. HIIT for beginners, like any other HIIT workout, is made up of five workouts – jumping jacks, burpees, squats, high knees, and raised arm cycles. Perform each of these workouts for 20 seconds to complete a circuit. Do five circuits with a 30 second rest after each.

2. You can do quick HIIT exercise anywhere

Morning is the perfect time to go HIITing for weight loss. Jumpstart your metabolism rate in the morning so you can burn more calories as you go through the rest of your day. A simple 3-exercise routine can give you a total body workout and burn a substantial number of calories. You can start with 15 reps of alternating spider climb, butterfly kicks, and a modified burpee. Repeat this circuit 3 times. You only need 15 to 20 minutes of this intensive workout.

3. 30-minute upper body HIIT workout

Streamline every muscle above your waist with this 30-minute HIIT exercise for the upper body muscles. This HIIT exercise targets the triceps, biceps, shoulders, and abs with six workouts divided into two circuits.

Start this exercise by warming up with cardio workouts. Then start with three rounds of circuit one – 12 reps of overhead press, chest press, and triceps kickback. Take a 30-second rest before walking one mile. After this, do three rounds of the second circuit – 12 reps of plank with lateral raise, 15 reps of triceps dip, and 15 reps of push-ups. Stretch to cool down.

4. 7-Move circuit

This workout boosts speed, strength, and fast metabolism. It is ideal for folks who are exercising for weight loss but are stuck on their weight plateau.

As the name indicates, the circuit is made up of 7

workouts – blast off, straight line lunge with circle pass, hero push up, twisted renegade, wipe and crush, armed warrior, and table hop. Repeat this circuit as many times as you can with one-minute rest between workouts.

5. 25-Minute total body HIIT

This workout requires yoga mats, dumbbells, and a small chair to perform. The 25-minute total body HIIT is made up of eight workouts – jump squats, squat press, glute bridges, push-ups, jumping jack, renegade rows, dips, and reverse crunches. Each workout is timed, and each circuit is designed to last 7.50 minutes. Performing 3 sets will result in a 25-minute complete body workout.

6. No equipment 30-minute HIIT exercise

This workout is made up of 8 exercises designed to target the body's major muscles. It comprises of lateral walking lunge, 180 squat jump, rolling forearm plank, push up with shoulder tap, inverted press, single leg glute bridge, bench V-sit up, and plyometric step up.

Set 40 seconds for each exercise and rest 10-20 seconds in between. Complete 3 rounds with 60-120 second rest between each round.

7. Incinerate body fat with high intensity circuit workout

This exercise is designed to maximize the afterburn, also known as Excess Post-Exposure Oxygen Consumption (EPOC). It is one of the most efficient ways of burning calories. By definition, afterburn is the amount of oxygen required to bring the body back to its normal metabolic function. Optimizing the afterburn effect is crucial if you want to sustain your weight loss.

This workout is made up of 12 exercises. Each exercise should take 30 seconds to perform. Set aside a 10-second rest before moving on to the next workout. Beginners should complete one round, intermediates 2-3 rounds, and advanced levels 3-4 rounds.

8. Body sculpting HIIT

This HIIT workout is made up of 12 exercises. You have the liberty to plan the number of reps and circuits you want to complete a round. Beginners can start with low reps and circuits before gradually increasing as you get used to the workout. To make your workout super effective, especially for weight loss purposes, just increase the number of circuits you can complete in a week.

9. HIIT the stairs

Doing HIIT on the stairs is total fun! All you need to do is find a long set of stairs and you will be good to go. This HIIT exercise is composed of 8 full-body exercises that you can do in and around the stairs. It is great if you do this exercise outdoors for a wider workout area and fresh air. Add fun and excitement to the workout by bringing friends along for the exercise.

10.   20-Minute HIIT workout

One of the simplest HIIT workouts recommended for beginners, the 21-Minute HIIT workout comprises of 5 exercises that you can do literally anywhere, even in your bedroom!

To get started, assign 45 seconds for each of the following exercises – side to side plank jumps, jump rope, alternating lunges with shoulder press, snowboarders, and in and out full-body crunches. Rest for 15 seconds after completing the circuit. Repeat this for 15-20 rounds.

Chapter 9: Sports and Weight Loss

If sport is your thing and you want to burn some calories, this is for you. Whether you are for team or individual sports, you should not have a problem finding a sport that causes some form of weight loss. Obviously, some sports will help you burn more fat than others. For better results, include at least 30 minutes of activity into your daily routine. You can do this all at once or break your workout into smaller segments through the day.

The 9 best sports that can accelerate your weight loss

Trying to burn calories? Here are the best and most fun sports that can help you realize your weight loss goals. And for most of them, you neither need expensive equipment nor costly monthly gym subscriptions.

To lose one pound per week, you will need to

burn about 3,500 calories. But it is important to understand that working out for hours is not all you need to lose weight – you also need to pay attention to your heart rate as well as the amount of effort you are putting into your activities. The maximum allowable heart rate you should hit is 220 less your age, but your target heart rate is what will get you in the calorie burning zone. Read below for an estimation of how many calories you can burn (when participating vigorously) in each activity for 30 minutes. Keep in mind that there may be a slight variation in your results

Individual sports

Swimming (Breaststroke):

460 calories per 30 active minutes in the water

Swimming is a cardio powerhouse that exercises the entire body. It is particularly great for those who want to benefit from low-impact exercise. You do not need a lot of equipment to get around this – just a swimsuit, goggles, and access to a swimming pool, of course. Of all the swimming styles, backstroke burns the most calories. You may also try front crawl or freestyle.

HIIT (High Intensity training sports)

450 calories per 30 minute activity

Technically, HIIT is not a sport per se. However, it is one of the best ways to burn calories and lose weight, and you can choose an activity based on the sports you play. As already discussed in previous chapters, HIIT is an exercise plan made up of repeated rounds of workouts performed at the maximum possible effort for a given time interval followed by short recovery periods. For instance, you could perform a minute of skater hops followed by 20 seconds of rest, followed by another minute of squats, and so on. The good news is, you do not need to buy anything for your HIIT workout.

Running

395 calories per 30 active minutes

Let's face it, all you need to run safely is a comfortable pair of running shoes, really. If you are new to running, try combining your running with walking sessions. If you are running to lose weight, be sure to check your heart rate and make sure that you are getting a rigorous workout. There are devices that you can use to monitor your heart rate while running as well as tally your steps as you run. You can also use applications to determine the distance you intend to run through as well as your effort and speed.

Rock climbing

330 calories per 30 active minutes

Rock climbing is a wonderful body weight resistance training workout. Of course, most folks find it intimidating to get started. However, you can start out at an indoor rock gym before taking your rock climbing venture outdoors. These gyms have basic equipment that can help you learn how to scale a rock wall – climbing shoes and a harness. They are also staffed with people with skills that can help you acquire vital skills for your venture.

Team sports for weight loss

Flag football

350 calories per 30 active minutes

Professional football may be littered with controversy, but flag football is quite safe and less likely to cause injury since it is a very little impact sport without painful tackling. Find a co-ed flag football team in your area. Most are designed for professionals in their 30s and 40s. Keep this in mind, though: as with every other team sport, its major downtimes are resting, waiting, or, in the case of football, huddling. As such, a 1-hour game might only provide you with 20-30 minutes of intensive movement.

Kickball

295 calories per 30 active minutes

Kickball tourneys are also fast growing in popularity, and just as with football, all you require as a comfortable pair of sport shoes and a set of play clothes. But again, there is a lot of downtime.

Zumba

270 calories per 30 active minutes

Again, Zumba is technically not a sport. However, it is an incredibly popular exercise class that is excellent for burning those extra calories. It is generally offered at fitness centers, but some will let you pay per class attended. To achieve success with Zumba for weight loss, you will need to put effort into mimicking your instructor's movements. Tip! If you are not sweating throughout the session, chances are you are not going to burn 270 calories at the end of the 30 minutes. The best part, however, is you will learn new dance moves for your next social gathering.

Basketball

(playing a game) 350 calories per 30 active minutes

Basketball (Shooting hoops) 175 calories per 30 active minutes

As you can see, you may play basketball as a team if you want to burn some calories and lose weight. The challenge of competing with another team will almost double your calorie burn. Most neighborhoods have free to access basketball courts, so all you need to do is dress up, put a team together, and hit the court. Tip! Always replace your shoes every six months if you are using them to exercise on a regular basis.

Chapter 10: Lifestyle adoption for weight loss, yoga, meditation, and Pilates.

Yoga and weight loss

Yoga exercise supports mental, physical, and spiritual development. The result is a better version of yourself.

But that is not all. Yoga can also help you lose weight, especially the more active versions of yoga. And you will realize that the awareness that comes with a gentle, relaxing yoga practice can greatly help you lose weight. Most experts agree that works in a different way to bring about a healthy weight. Let us look at a few of these ways.

Yoga and Mindfulness

Yoga's spiritual and mental aspects are geared towards developing mindfulness. This boosts your awareness on many levels. It will increase your consciousness on how different foods affect your body, mind, and spirit. According to a 2016 study, folks who develop mindfulness through yoga are best placed to say no to unhealthy foods and eating habits. They are also likely to become more in tune with their bodies so that they can notice when they have had enough.

Yoga is believed to be especially beneficial for folks who are struggling with weight loss through other approaches as well.

According to a 2017 study, mindfulness training can have a positive short-term benefit when it comes to binge or impulsive eating as well as participation in physical activities that facilitate weight loss. While the study did not find a direct link between mindfulness and weight loss, experts believe weight loss is associated with extended periods of mindfulness training. Certainly, more study is needed to expand on these findings.

Since practicing yoga on a full stomach is not

advisable, you are likely to find yourself making healthy eating decisions before doing yoga. After your yoga session, you are likely to crave fresh, unprocessed foods. Most folks also learn to chew each bite more thoroughly and eat slowly, which can result in less food intake.

Yoga and better sleep

Regular yoga practice can improve the quality of your sleep. You may learn that you are able to fall asleep with ease, and sleep deeply, when you have a consistent yoga exercise. Ideally, you need six to nine hours of sleep.

Studies have linked quality sleep with weight loss. According to a 2018 study by Oxford Academic, people who had restricted sleep five times a week burnt less fat than those who stuck with their regular sleep patterns. Both groups limited the number of calories they consumed, indicating that lack of sleep adversely affects the body's composition, including weight loss.

Yoga nidra is a guided relaxation that you practice while lying down. The practice has been found to help improve sleep and increase an individual's mindfulness. During your yoga nindra session, you may set intentions that can help you realize your weight loss goals.

Another 2018 study by Ovid found that healthcare workers who routinely practiced yoga nidra for eight weeks had an improved level of mindfulness. This mindfulness included acting with extreme awareness while not judging their inner experiences.

Yoga and calorie burning

Of course, yoga is not your traditional aerobic exercise. That said, it is important to understand that some yoga types are more physical than others.

And active, intense forms of yoga can definitely help you burn some calories. This can help keep weight gain at bay. Vinyasa, Ashtanga, and power yoga are examples of physical yoga that can help you burn calories and lose weight.

Vinyasa and power yoga are usually available at the hot yoga studios. These forms of yoga keep you in motion almost constantly, which in turn helps you burn fat.

Consistent yoga practice may also help you tone your muscles and improve your metabolism.

While restorative yoga is not a physical type of yoga, it can still help you lose weight. A study by AJMC found that restorative yoga can help overweight women to burn abdominal fat and lose weight. These finding are quite promising especially for folks whose body weight make more physical forms of yoga challenging.

Finally, a 2013 study concluded that yoga is a promising way to address weight loss, behavioral change, and maintenance by burning calories, reducing stress, and improving mindfulness. These factors can help you in managing your food intake and gaining awareness of the effects of overeating.

So how often should you practice yoga for weight loss?

It is advisable that you practice yoga as often as possible in order to lose weight. You may opt for a more physical, active form of yoga at least 3-5 times per week for at least an hour. On the other days, consider balancing your practice with a more gentle, relaxing form of yoga. Great options include yin, hatha, and restorative yoga.

If you are a beginner, it is advisable that you start early before consistently building up your practice. This allows you to consolidate your strength and flexibility while preventing injuries. If you are unable to get time for full time classes on certain days, try out a self-practice for at least 30 minutes. Set aside one full day for rest each week.

For better weight loss results, it is best when you combine your yoga practice with activities like cycling, walking, and swimming for additional cardiovascular benefits.

As part of your routine, do not weigh yourself immediately after your yoga classes, especially if you are from a hot yoga class since you may lose some weight during the session. Instead, set aside some time each day to weigh yourself.

Best yoga poses for weight loss

Here are a few yoga poses that you can practice at home if you do not have the time for a full yoga class.

Sun salutations

Practice at least 10 Sun Salutations. You may adjust the intensity by holding some of the positions for extended periods or by speeding up the pace.

1. From a standing position, breathe in as you lift your arms overhead

2. Breathe out as you swan dive down into a forward bend position

3. Jump, step, or walk your feet back into a plank position

4. Remain in this position for five breaths

5. While dropping your knee down, lower your body to the floor

6. Spread your legs, turn your feet tops to the mat and place your hands under your shoulders

7. Breathe in to lift partway, halfway, or all the way up for a cobra pose

8. Breathe out to lower your back down and then push up into a downward facing dog

9. Remain in this pose for five breaths

10. Breathe out as you jump, step, or walk your feet to the top of the mat and stand in forward bend

11. Then breathe in to lift your arms over your head

12. Breathe out to lower your arms back down by your body

Boat pose

This pose engages the entire body, with special focus on the core, and can help reduce your stress levels.

1. Sit on your yoga mat with your legs together and extended in front of you

2. While bending your knees, lift your feet off the floor so your thighs are at an angle to the floor while your shins are parallel to the floor.

3. Raise your arms in front of you to a parallel position with the floor

4. Straighten your legs, if you can, while keeping your torso in a lifted position

5. Remain in this position for 30 seconds

6. Repeat 5-6 times

Plank pose

You can spend 10-20 minutes doing various variations of this pose

1. From the tabletop position, step your feet back while lifting your heels

2. Align your body into a straight line. You may want the help of a mirror to get into this position

3. Get your core, leg, and arm muscles engaged

4. Remain in this position for at least 5 minutes

Meditation and weight loss

Meditation is the practice of clearing one's mind by closing one's eyes and focusing on your breathing for the purpose of having one's emotions and thinking calm and straightforward.

Some experts have suggested that meditating daily for between 10 to 20 minutes is ideal.

However, for beginners, meditation can last for up to 5 minutes since adapting to a new routine can be challenging. You can start by meditating every morning immediately after you wake up. The first few times will be challenging since your mind will keep wandering, but be focused and determined.

For maximum benefits and for it to be effective, meditation has to be done regularly and in a comfortable setting. Depending on what is more comfortable for you, you can either meditate while sitting or lying down.

What's the connection between meditation and weight loss?

Since meditation involves the mind, it has been regarded as an effective weight loss tool. The conscious mind is the main controller of our behavior and habits formed or acquired from our unconscious mind. These include habits like stress eating and craving for foods that are unhealthy which are some of the causes of weight gain. Meditation aligns our mind, both conscious and unconscious, to agree on the necessary changes that one wants to make to our habits and behaviors. These include controlling our cravings and instead introducing healthy eating habits.

Cortisol is a hormone that helps the body in responding to stress. Experts say that when stressed, it causes calories to be stored as fat in the body. This means that no matter how healthy one eats, high stress levels will make you add weight. Daily meditation has been known to reduce the level of stress by calming the body and mind. It mostly affects the conscious mind which is the part of the brain that controls what we do. That means you can see a jar of cookies and have the willpower to pass it.

How can meditation help when diet and exercise don't seem to be working?

Stress has been known to be one of the major causes of weight gain. You have been faithful to your exercising routine and diet yet your weight keeps going up. The lack of positive results in your weight loss routine will add more stress, hence you end up adding more weight instead of losing it. Remember, more stress = more hormones = more fat. Meditation together with the weight loss routine is the best way to lose weight.

For a start, identify the source of your stress. To do this, experts have developed gadgets such as the WellBe. It is a bracelet which will help you in identifying the stress triggers in your day to day activities as it focuses on your emotional state. This way you can easily develop habits and routines that will help you in your weight loss.

Another way is to note down every time you are stressed and what stressed you. You can do the same with the food that you eat. This way you will learn to avoid situations that will develop into stress and thus making you to revert to your old ways. You will also learn how to manage stressful situations with the breathing in and breathing out exercise. This may take less than 5 minutes of your time even if you are at work which means you can even have a quick meditation over your lunch break.

How can you make sure meditation works for you?

As earlier mentioned, meditation works best when it is practiced as a daily routine in a comfortable and stress-free environment. There are ways you can include meditation in your daily routine without it being a bother. Remember, it's here to reduce your stress not be a source of stress. Here are a few tips on how to use meditation without it being a bother:

Use a mantra that helps you lose weight. When meditating, you may need a word or a phrase that will keep your mind from wandering. That's a mantra. It is not a must that you have one if it will not be helpful or if it feels forced. However if you decide to have one, repeat it when you inhale and when you exhale. If you choose not to have a mantra, just meditate normally by just focusing on your breathing

Follow your breath to reduce stress. Meditation is all about reducing stress levels and calming you down. Holding your breath when you exhale and inhale helps in calming one down and it reduces stress. Experts suggest using a four count and eight count when inhaling and exhaling respectively. If it doesn't come naturally, don't force it. If you force it the meditation will end up being your source of distress and not calmness. Take it one step at a time. You can start from one and move upwards. Note that having a long exhale calms you significantly.

Try a guided meditation for weight loss.

Maybe you feel like you do not understand all that you have read about meditation or you do not feel motivated when doing the meditation alone? Not to worry. There are resources on the world wide web that will guide you up to a point where you're comfortable enough to try it on your own.

There is also the option of establishments which offer meditation classes for a large group of people. You can enroll in one of these and have the motivation that you need.

What should you expect from doing guided meditation for weight loss?

Remember not all meditations lead to weight loss. If you are meditating specifically to assist you in weight loss, look for resources that deal specifically with weight loss. You will find experts who have used meditation to lose weight and this will be an inspiration to your cause. You will learn how to include the weight loss regime in your daily routine, how to lose and keep the weight off.

Are there limitations to using meditation techniques for weight loss?

There are no limitations to using meditation for weight loss. However, it is important to note that this is just one of the three parts to a successful weight loss regime. You have to fully incorporate the diet and exercise part of it and be dedicated and consistent to the entire routine. Experts have proven that meditation when practiced for a period of 21 days alters the structure of the brain. It is advisable to get a routine that you can continue in the long-term and not one that stresses you.

Meditation techniques for weight loss

There are several techniques that are good for any weight loss enthusiast. Followed diligently and combined with a balanced diet and cardio exercise, you will have a lean toned body and will have lost significant weight in no time. Below are a few techniques that will be of benefit to your weight loss routine:

1. Dumbbell Squat, 3 minutes

Hold both the dumbbells in both hands by the side of your hips. Keep your feet slightly apart with your toes straight and your back upright.

Start squatting while spreading your knees apart and your back upright. Do 3 to 4 reps every 10 seconds and repeat for 3 minutes. Your heart rate should be below 150bpm through the entire exercise.

2. TRX Inverted Row, 2 minutes per session

Pick TRX straps from underneath with your feet drawn together to the anchor point. Raise your shoulder blades together and lift yourself while keeping your body in a plank position. Repeat this exercise 2 to 3 reps for up to two minutes – keep your heart rate below 150 bpm during the workout period.

3. 3 chin-up reps

Grab a pull-up bar with your palm in an inward direction and start lifting your shoulder blades. Lift yourself up, leading towards your chest.

4. Arm Waiter's Walk, 20 yards each arm

Hold both dumbbells in both hands and walk. Repeat exercise for 30 minutes.

Chapter 11: Pilates and weight loss

What is Pilates?

Pilates is a form of weight loss regime which exercises the body and mind to achieve the optimum results. The connection of the mind and body is crucial for the success of Pilates

Pilates is a form of exercise that focuses on using both the mind and body to achieve optimum performance. The deep stabilizing muscles of the body are conditioned and strengthened using sequences of movements that use gravity, body weight, and specially designed equipment as forms of resistance. The connection between the mind and body is crucial to Pilates. Pilates trains the mind to maintain a constant level of awareness of the way the body moves. This results in a greater control of motion and vastly improved technique.

The History of Pilates

Joseph Pilates (1912-1967) developed Pilates regime of exercises to overcome the weaknesses he had as a child which included asthma, rheumatic fever, and rickets. It has become the best way for rehabilitating and rejuvenating the body. Joseph Pilates worked with war veterans from World War 1 who were paralyzed due to the injuries they suffered.

Benefits of Pilates

- Total Body Workout

Pilates works the whole body with each muscle in unison. Pilates prepares your body to handle daily physical challenges.

- Core Stability & Postural Alignment

Since Pilates gives the whole body a total workout, and all muscles work in unison, the body will always have a proper posture even in movement. This makes the chance of getting exhaustion or injury due to overuse of one area less. It also reduces body pains and aches related to bad posture.

- Muscle Tone and Strength

In order for Pilates to be effective and for you to achieve the desired effects, you should have one session on a daily basis and a 30-minute cardiovascular workout. This will make you have sculptured muscles and greatly reduce a high percentage of body fat in your body.

The PM's workouts consist of Pilates and regular jogging sessions; this is a great combination. Pilates isn't a cardiovascular workout and will not exercise your heart and lungs enough to reduce your chances of developing heart disease.

- Improved Body Awareness

Pilates workouts are designed to improve balance and coordination by teaching a greater connection between the mind and body. Many older clients that I have trained have forgotten how to use various muscles and their reaction times are slow. This is often very frustrating for them and it comes as a surprise. Pilates is an ideal way to get back in touch with your own body so that you can use it to its full potential.

- Injury Rehabilitation

Pilates' greatest benefit is that it is a low impact form of exercise thus making it the best when it comes to physical therapy. It rebuilds the strength and functionality of the injured parts of the body.

Just as Pilates is not a substitute for medicine, the exercise is also for you to do. You have to combine the medication prescribed and advice given by your doctor together with Pilates to achieve maximum results. It gives you the choice to take control of improving yourself. For assistance there are several sites that have private instructors who will help you through the routine in a safe way. In case you have any injuries, consult with your doctor before embarking on the Pilates exercising routine.

- Pilates for Weight Loss

Pilates burns calories depending on the intensity of your regime and, the more calories you burn, the more weight you will lose. The best way to achieve good results is by combining Pilates with a 30-minute cardiovascular exercise routine daily. Pilates makes the body stronger with each passing day.

Pilates gives a confidence boost which means less stress, thus reduced fat storage in the body.

- *Stress Reduction.*

Pilates helps in regulating your breathing which helps in stress reduction. When you're performing your Pilates, you are mostly focused on your movement and breathing. This allows you to push all the stressful thoughts to the back of your mind. When the exercise is done, you will come out more calm and fit to face the voices in your head with a clear mind.

Different variations of Pilates

Stott Pilates

Stott Pilates is the most recent form of Pilates in comparison to the rest. It has been revised by experts to conform to the latest forms of rehabilitation. This Pilates is good and appropriate for everyone. The sale of equipment as well of training of the instructors is carried out by the Stott Pilate Company.

Body Control Pilates®

The Body Control type of Pilates is for anyone with any form of injury. It has become a favorite with most osteopaths who are increasingly recommending it for rehabilitation purposes for most of their patients.

This workout is based on the following eight principles:

- Alignment
- Relaxation

- Centering: creating a strong girdle
- Breathing
- Coordination
- Stamina
- Flowing movements

Body Balance

Body Balance is a class found in most gyms countrywide. It is a made up of a combination of yoga, Tai Chi, and Pilates. This class is ideal for the contemporary style enthusiasts who are looking for something dynamic and modern. You can check online to find a class near you.

Pilates Equipment

Mat Work Classes

These classes are more widely available than the apparatus class because it only requires a mat unlike the apparatus class which has more equipment. Sometimes balls and resistance bands are used in this class. The main exercises in this class include helping the body to work against gravity. This class is best recommended for people who are beginners in Pilates. This will help them in getting acquainted with the basic level of stability before they can graduate to apparatus class which has more equipment to work with.

Who is Pilates Good For?

Pilates does not have a particular clientele. It is for everyone who has the dedication and desire. Everyone wants to have a good physique that is the envy of others. We would appreciate it even more if they would be stable enough to not get unnecessary avoidable injuries.

Does it work?

Everyone has a different body and different exercise routines work for different people in different ways depending on their aim for the exercise. The best way to know if it works is to give it a try and be dedicated and focused. Pilates is always being updated with the latest information

Pilates versus Yoga

Even though both of them work on the body and mind, there is a very small difference between Pilates and yoga. Pilates is more on the physical side while yoga is more on the spiritual side.

If you need a strong, lean physique and rehabilitation from injury then Pilates is for you, if you are looking for spirituality relaxation then yoga is for you.

How to Start Pilates Classes

The cost of classes differs depending on which one you sign up for and they are well structured. You can either sign up for the mat or apparatus sessions. The group mat sessions cost between $10-$15 while the group apparatus classes cost between $18 and $45. You may contact your local leisure center to find out if this program is available in your area.

One to One Sessions

This class is the best because the instructor only concentrates on you. This class is recommended for pregnant women, or anyone with an injury that needs full physical therapy. Although this class is slightly expensive (between $18 and $45), it is convenient in that you can either go to the class or the instructor can come to a place of your convenience.

Teach Yourself Pilates

The best part about teaching yourself Pilates is that you learn at your own pace and at your own convenience. There are shops, either online or in the streets, that sell books and DVDs that have step by step instructions on how to teach yourself. Each session goes at your own pace too, making it possible for you to refer back to what you did not get.

Is Pilates a good exercise for weight loss?

As much as Pilates is good for toning the body and muscle building, its effectiveness as a weight loss routine is not so much. This is due to the fact that it is an exercise that does not involve intense exercise unlike swimming and jogging. This means that you burn fewer calories. However, it will help you in attaining a healthy weight and live a healthy lifestyle.

For weight loss, Pilates has to be combined with strength and cardio exercise routines and a healthy diet. The routines should be done in alternation.

Read on to learn more about the benefits of Pilates and the role it can play in helping you to lose weight.

How many calories does Pilates burn?

Your current weight and the difficulty of the class you are taking will determine how many calories you will burn. For instance, a 150 pound adult can burn 175 calories with a 50-minute exercise.

To achieve maximum calorie loss, it is advisable to take the reformer class or be in a class where your heart rate is elevated.

How do calories affect weight loss?

A single pound is equivalent to 3500 calories. This means that if you burn 3500 calories, you have lost one pound. This is a guide for you to know how many pounds you are losing in any exercise you undertake. In addition, a healthy diet should be included in the routine.

How often should you practice Pilates?

As a beginner, people tend to overindulge in anything we do. The same happens to exercise. Beginners are advised to start with a routine of 3 to 5 times a week.

Once you have gone past the 21 day routine and your body is accustomed to the routine, you may move to the more advanced classes. These classes will make you burn more calories.

Do not forget to alternate between eating a

healthy diet, Pilates, strength and cardio exercises to tone your body and help you to reach your weight targets in your weight loss routines.

If you're trying to lose weight, participate in these types of combination classes a few times a week for the best results. You can also alternate Pilates classes with strength training sessions (with weights) and cardio exercise.

What is the Pilates effect?

The "Pilates effect" is the belief that one has lost weight and toned specific parts of their body due to their practicing Pilates.

This makes you look fit even in cases where you haven't lost any weight.

Tips for weight loss

- Keep in mind that no routine works alone. You have to exercise and eat a balanced diet to achieve the best results.

- Your meals must be inclusive of all the

nutrients.

- Your daily food consumption must contain more than 1,200 calories.

Conclusion

Obesity is an epidemic in the developed world. The number of overweight and obese Americans, for instance, is growing at an alarming rate, especially in recent years. In fact, some studies claim that over 60 percent of Americans are now considered overweight, with about 30 percent of Americans considered to be obese.

These numbers represent a tragic public health story. Being overweight can increase your risk of lifestyle illnesses like diabetes, cardiovascular problems, and some forms of cancers. Healthy weight management has nothing to with slim-down shakes or miracle pills. Rather, it takes work, time, and commitment. As already established, the weight you are trying to lose did not show up overnight, and it is certainly going to take time to burn off. A healthy pace of weight loss is about 1-2 pounds per week. The rewards of a healthy lifestyle change can be phenomenal, with its effects on different aspects of your life.

Making a conscious decision to embrace a healthy lifestyle will not just help you fit those skinny jeans: it will also let you set a great example for your kids that they can follow into adulthood. It will help you have a positive outlook as you go about your daily routines. It will equip you with the endurance you need to do the things you love for longer without running out of energy. It will boost your mood and self-esteem. And yes, it will save you money.

www.ingramcontent.com/pod-product-compliance
Lightning Source LLC
Chambersburg PA
CBHW031147020426
42333CB00013B/549